SECRETS OF THE LEAN PLATE CLUB

Secrets of

THE LEAN PLATE CLUB

A Simple Step-by-Step Program
to Help You Shed Pounds and
Keep Them Off for Good

SALLY SQUIRES, M.S.

ST. MARTIN'S PRESS ✹ NEW YORK

www.stmartins.com

Library of Congress Cataloging-in-Publication Data

Squires, Sally.
    Secrets of the Lean Plate Club : a simple step-by-step program to help you shed pounds and keep them off for good / Sally Squires.
        p.   cm.
Includes index.
ISBN 0-312-33917-8
EAN 978-0-312-33917-3
1. Reducing diets.   2. Weight loss.   I. Title.

RM222.2.S72   2006
613.2'5—dc22

                                                                    2005057439

First Edition: April 2006

10   9   8   7   6   5   4   3   2   1

To my family, especially John, Colin, Ian, and my father, who cheered me on every step of the way, and to sweet Cafall and Cutter, for sharing their lives with us and getting us to move more

A NOTE TO READERS

CONTENTS

ACKNOWLEDGMENTS

No book is done in a vacuum. While an author's name goes beneath the title, many participate in a book's publication in a variety of ways. *Washington Post* Health Editor Craig Stoltz gave me the freedom and the encouragement to create and nurture this bold, new venture, enabling the Lean Plate Club to grow into an online community and nationally syndicated column. Every reporter should be so lucky.

To the many experts—scientists, registered dietitians, physicians, and other health professionals—who regularly find time to answer my questions, put up with calls at inconvenient hours, and send scientific papers, thank you. I am forever grateful for your help. I'd especially like to thank Kathryn McMurry, Ph.D., at the U.S. Department of Health and Human Services Office of Disease Prevention and Health Promotion, as well as Lorelei DiSogra, R.D., former head of the National Cancer Institute's 5 to 9 a Day program. At the U.S. Department of Agriculture, grateful thanks go as well to Eric Hentges, Ph.D., and his staff at the Center for Nutrition Policy and Promotion, and to Shanthy Bowman, Ph.D., of the USDA's Agricultural Research Service. All these dedicated public servants have patiently answered my many questions about the latest Dietary Guidelines, the Food Guide Pyramid, and many other related subjects too numerous to list here. Any misinterpretations included in this volume are mine alone.

At *The Washington Post,* washingtonpost.com, and the *Washington Post* Writer's Group, a team of people have enabled the Lean Plate Club to thrive. Special thanks go to Leonard Downie, Phil Bennett, Alan Shearer, James Hill, Michael Keegan, Eric Lieberman, Jim Brady, Doug Feaver, Ju-Don Marshall Roberts, Stacey Palosky, Liz Kelly, Katie McLeod, Sarah Lumbard, Laura Cochran, Jennifer Lilly, Linda Haskins-Wrenn, Rodney Johnson, Karisue Wyson, Jennifer Ferrell, Karen Greene, Richard Aldacushion, Greg Mott, Tom Graham, Susan Morse, Lisa Schreiber, Eric Grant, and Lisa Bolton, and to Stacie Reistetter, John Nichols, and Eleanor Hong, who helped nurture the early Lean Plate Club but have now moved on to new ventures outside the *Post.*

Two *Washington Post* colleagues deserve very special recognition and thanks: Patterson Clark, who created the exercise drawings in this book, and Randall Mays, who designed the first Lean Plate Club logo and illustrated many of the early columns.

Literary agent Marcy Posner believed in this project from the beginning and shepherded it to St. Martin's Press, where Diane Reverand, Regina Scarpa, and Frances Sayers have smoothly guided it to publication.

Finally, this book would not exist without the growing community of loyal Lean Plate Club members, who, in our weekly Web chats, graciously help one another and prove by example that it is possible to eat smart and move more to reach a healthier weight. They provide continual inspiration to us all.

INTRODUCTION

"I don't know what to eat!" is a complaint I hear repeatedly from people of all ages, sexes, and shapes in my job writing the "Lean Plate Club" column at *The Washington Post.* "Should I follow South Beach or Weight Watchers? And what's the best way to work out, especially if I hate to exercise?"

Despite our best public health efforts, a multibillion-dollar weight-loss industry, the sale of millions of diet books—some 35 million of South Beach and Atkins alone—and the high-profile weight struggles of Oprah, Sarah Ferguson, and Al Roker, the nation isn't getting thinner. It's getting fatter.

Look around. Two out of every three Americans weigh too much. Forty-four million people are at least 30 pounds or more above their healthy weight, placing them roundly in the ranks of the obese. Another 123 million are overweight and headed for obesity if they don't do something to stop it.

All these extra pounds take a significant health toll. Weight-related diseases now cost more than $200 billion annually in medical treatment and lost productivity. How many people die from being too fat is under debate, but the latest estimates from the federal Centers for Disease Control and Prevention suggest that about 100,000 people die prematurely each year because of weight-related illnesses.

Obesity also fuels heart disease, cancer, stroke, and diabetes—

four of the top ten causes of death in the United States. A 2004 *Time*/ABC News poll showed that 58 percent of Americans would like to lose weight, nearly twice the percentage who felt that way in 1951, but only 27 percent said they were trying to slim down—and two-thirds of those weren't following any specific plan to do so.

It sounds hopeless, but it's not.

On July 29, 2001, I started the "Lean Plate Club" column in the *Washington Post* "Health" section and began hosting a weekly Web chat by the same name at www.washingtonpost.com. In 2002, we launched a companion Lean Plate Club e-mail newsletter.

The "Lean Plate Club" column is now nationally syndicated and read weekly by millions of people from coast to coast. Each Tuesday, the Lean Plate Club Web chat draws participants from Boston to Los Angeles, and internationally from as far away as Turkey, Spain, Scotland, Australia, Colombia, Japan, and India. Nearly 250,000 people also subscribe to the weekly Lean Plate Club e-mail newsletter, and the numbers continue to grow. Throughout the world, Lean Plate Club "members" say that they are enjoying food again for the first time in a long time. Many report significant results from their new lifestyles. They are losing weight and feel better for doing so.

By following the *Secrets of the Lean Plate Club,* you're joining tens of thousands of people who are giving up dieting and deprivation and learning how to *add*—yes, you read that right—great-tasting, healthful food and more physical activity to their lives to achieve a healthier weight. And they are doing it without special foods, weight-loss medications, or weight-loss surgery.

Secrets of the Lean Plate Club will help you determine what works best for you to achieve a healthier weight. Losing weight is, of course, only half the battle. Keeping it off is key. Unless you learn to change the habits that allowed your unwanted pounds to pile on in the first place, you are doomed to fail. That's where the

Lean Plate Club philosophy comes in. It teaches you how to change your habits. For good.

During the next eight weeks on the Lean Plate Club Program, you'll learn what Lean Plate Club members have learned and are putting into practice. Using simple, step-by-step instructions, you'll find out how to eat smart and move more, no matter how busy or unpredictable your schedule. There are no forbidden foods, no complicated formulas, and no guilt on the Lean Plate Club. It's all about rediscovering the joy of savoring great-tasting, healthful food and finding ways to be more physically active every day.

Here's the real Lean Plate Club advantage: Whether you strictly follow the eight-week program included in these pages or adhere to Atkins or Weight Watchers, South Beach or Dean Ornish, Fat Flush, the G.I. Diet, Volumetrics, Dr. Phil's Ultimate Weight Solution, Carbo Addicts, Eat for Life, the L.A. Shape Diet, Jenny Craig, the Perfect Fit Diet, the Food Doctor Diet, the Abs Diet, the Maker's Diet, Sugar Busters, the Okinawa Diet, Jorge Cruise's 3-Hour Diet, the French Women Don't Get Fat approach, the Zone, or any other weight-loss plan, the Lean Plate Club philosophy can supercharge any of them. Or be used alone.

You'll also find the social support, tips, and inspiration that Lean Plate Club members share with one another online in the weekly Web chat or read in my free weekly e-mail newsletter. This resource combination has earned the Lean Plate Club special recognition from the Society of Public Health Educators, the American Society of Clinical Nutrition, and the American Society for Nutrition. The Lean Plate Club has also been named a model program by the Rails to Trails Conservancy in a booklet sponsored by the Robert Wood Johnson Foundation.

The eight-week program included in this book is flexible and simple. Each week, you'll find two new goals—one for food and one for activity. The Lean Plate Club Program helps you put into practice the most up-to-date nutritional advice. Plus, you don't have to pay to attend group meetings. Nowhere in the Lean Plate Club will you suffer from harsh bullying, scolding, or guilt. It's a commonsense, back-to-basics approach that will help you control your eating once and for all. Not only will you feel better, but the Lean Plate Club also shows you how to savor a wide variety of healthy foods that fad diets don't allow. And it will teach you how to build more exercise into your daily life by doing the physical activity that you enjoy most.

Finally, you get me: a nationally known, award-winning medical writer for *The Washington Post,* whose beat is nutrition. (You can reach me anytime via e-mail at leanplateclub@washpost.com. I read all my messages and respond personally to as many as time allows.) I also talk daily with the world's leading nutrition and exercise experts. Plus, I've got the educational background—a master's degree in nutrition from Columbia University's Institute of Human Nutrition and another master's from Columbia's Graduate School of Journalism—to dig deeply into the scientific literature and make sense of the conflicting nutrition and exercise information that bombards you day after day.

And yes, I know personally about weight struggles. Despite having a graduate degree in nutrition, I, too, have experienced how a sedentary, stressful, and busy life can pile on the pounds when you're not paying attention. I know about waging the battle of the bulge. Most of us can't afford to hire a personal trainer and a chef to help control our weight. Let's note that even famous movie stars with unlimited resources and much more flexible schedules than most of us still have to work very hard to keep their weight under control. No wonder the rest of us need extra assistance to stay on track.

Part One

THE BASICS

One

SECRETS OF
THE LEAN PLATE CLUB

The messages often begin like this:

> "Hi, Sally. I need to lose 20 pounds for a wedding later this month. What can I do?"

> "Dear Sally—I've lost 35 pounds over the past year, but now I find that I'm slipping into my old eating habits, and I just can't find the motivation to exercise. Help! I don't want to put this weight back on after I worked so hard to take it off."

> "Hey, Sally. I just got on the scale and I can't believe what I weigh! I don't know how this happened. Where do I start?"

> "Sally—I'm working in my first job. I know I've been partying a little on the weekends, but the pounds are just piling on. If it's like this now, what's it going to be like when I'm 30?"

> "Sally, I've lost 25 pounds in the last six months, but my weight seems to have plateaued for the last few weeks. I am so discouraged. What do I do now?"

You can feel the frustration, impatience, and desperation in these messages. There's a sense of being out of control. Behind many of them is the nagging, unspoken fear that often comes wrapped in a little bit of panic: "Maybe I can't take the weight off. Maybe this really is hopeless."

I'm here to tell you that it's not.

Lean Plate Club members prove that week after week. Will the pounds melt away? Nope, I can't promise that. Successful weight loss takes time, focus, and commitment. Anybody who tells you otherwise is not being honest. And yes, the majority of people do experience a discouraging weight plateau somewhere in the process. But there are easy steps to make this a simpler journey, one that you can enjoy. Just ask Melissa Glassman, 50, who with help from the Lean Plate Club has lost half her body weight, going from 250 pounds on a 5'3" frame to a healthy 125 pounds. Whether you are trying to hold the line on future weight gain, shed a few pounds, or make some major changes like Melissa, the lessons in *Secrets of the Lean Plate Club* can help you achieve your goals.

Since I began the Lean Plate Club in July 2001, I've interviewed hundreds of experts, read several thousand pages of scientific journals, and been in contact with tens of thousands of Lean Plate Club members by e-mail, via the Web chat, and by phone. So to whet your soon-to-be-healthier appetite, here are just some of the secrets that you'll find in the pages ahead. Knowing and practicing these secrets will help you to reach a healthier weight and live like a thinner person.

Calories *do* count. Forget all the hype and empty promises. Yes, it does come down to the numbers: calories in versus calories out. Eat too much, burn too few calories, and the pounds add up—whether you adhere to a low-fat regimen, eliminate carbohydrates, or become a vegetarian. It doesn't matter. You're going to have to change the numbers in your favor, which means a deficit of daily calories to lose weight.

Amherst Mass.: Hi, Sally! Since I've lost 64 pounds, people often ask what the secret is. Well guess what? It's measuring portion sizes, knowing what a portion is, tracking food for the day, and exercising more. Recently, I hit a plateau and wondered why. I realized I'd been guessing in my head instead of writing down the number of servings in each food group every day. So the dreaded "calorie creep" happened. Three days after resuming keeping a little chart—which only takes a minute—I lost two more pounds and have continued that way to reach a body mass index of 21.9, down from 30.

"But what about Atkins or South Beach? They don't count calories." Read the fine print, and you'll find that some form of calorie restriction is part of every well-known weight-loss plan from Atkins to the Zone. That's why in a few pages, you'll discover how to calculate the right number of daily calories for you, including so-called discretionary calories for indulging in such treats as a glass of a wine or a piece of chocolate.

Diets don't work long-term. On the weekly Lean Plate Club Web chat, I've jokingly said that I could develop the Whipped Cream Diet and guarantee that it would produce weight loss. At least for a while. That's because virtually every diet does work in the short term. The simple act of monitoring what you eat automatically helps you focus on and decrease how many calories you consume. Cut calories and the weight starts to come off.

I can also guarantee that there would come a time when the novelty of eating whipped cream every day would wear off. In fact, you'd eventually get sick of whipped cream. Then you'd add back the other foods that the Whipped Cream Diet eliminated to keep calories in check. As you can probably guess, you'd start regaining weight, which is what happens with every other diet. They all stop working, because they're too restrictive, too complicated, or both. Pretty soon boredom sets in, nutritional mischief follows, and . . . well, you know the rest. To succeed, you must find a way of eating and staying active that you can live with long-term. For one 45-year-old Lean Plate Club member and his wife, that means establishing an exercise room in their basement, setting aside time for early-morning walks together, and making more of their food from scratch so that they can control calories and avoid processed ingredients.

You didn't put on the weight overnight. It may seem like rolls of fat have suddenly padded your waist, derriere, thighs, arms, back, chest, and stomach, but unwanted pounds creep on slowly and insidiously. Just an extra 100 calories per day—less than the amount found in a grande skim latte or a candy bar—add up to an extra ten pounds per year. Ten pounds this year, ten pounds next, and it's no longer a mystery why you, along with two-thirds of the U.S. adult population, have a lot of unwanted weight to lose. There are no quick fixes for these extra pounds, but the good news is that by making some simple habit changes, the odds are good that you can lose the weight in a fraction of the time that you gained it.

There is no one way to achieve a healthy weight. Numerous diet books and commercial weight-loss plans claim to provide the "right way" to lose weight, but there's no scientific evidence to back those claims. Every diet works for someone, at least temporarily. No diet works for everyone. During the Lean Plate Club Program, you'll add at least one healthy habit weekly—sometimes more—that will slowly, but steadily, help you to achieve a healthier weight. Think of it as attention to behavior change or the ABCs of the Lean Plate Club philosophy. By tailoring healthy eating to your food preferences and the kind of physical activity you like best to your daily schedule, you'll develop healthier habits for good. Anyone can do drastic things to reach a goal weight temporarily. But unless you eat what you like and do something you enjoy to work out, odds are that you won't stick with any drastic measures for long, and the weight will return.

If you have:	Switch to:	Save:
Once weekly		
Two-scoop ice-cream cone	single-dip cone	115 calories each
Do that for a year = nearly 2 pounds lost		
Three times weekly		
Mocha Frappuccino	grande cappuccino	190 calories each
(grande, 16 ounces)	with skim milk	
Do that for a year = potentially 8 pounds lost		
Five times weekly		
1 ounce potato chips	1 ounce pretzels	352 calories each
Do that for a year = about 4 pounds lost		

Small changes have big rewards. For some 48 million Americans, only about 20 pounds stand between them and a healthier body weight. It's very easy to replace high-calorie fare with a few lower-calorie foods and reap significant weight-loss benefits.

Doing the math helps. One pound is equivalent to 3,500 calories. If you want to lose 20 pounds, you need to "lose" 70,000 calories ($20 \times 3,500 = 70,000$). Daunting as that may sound, spread those 70,000 calories over the next 365 days ($70,000 \div 365 = 192$) to see that it takes a mere deficit of 192 calories daily to achieve a 20-pound weight loss in just one year. While that isn't a quick weight loss, losing weight slowly but steadily means that you are more apt to keep off the pounds.

How easy is it to trim calories with smart swaps? This easy: Substitute a glass of skim for 2 percent milk and save 42 calories. If you drink three glasses of milk daily—the goal of the latest U.S. Dietary Guidelines—that adds up to a savings of 126 calories per day. Over the course of a year, it could equal a 13-pound weight loss.

Or trade your super-size fries (610 calories) for small fries (210 calories) and cut 400 calories. Do that just once a week, and in nine weeks you could lose one pound. Switch from a one-ounce bag of potato chips daily to a one-ounce bag of pretzels and trim 52 calories per day—the equivalent of four pounds over a year. Drink a 12-ounce can of diet soda instead of regular to save 140 calories. Do that five times per week and it could add up to a ten-pound loss per year.

The right carbs are a good thing. In fact, without them, your brain may not get the fuel that it needs daily, and you could be missing out on key vitamins, minerals, and other health-promoting phytonutrients, not to mention fiber. Oh yes, and there's great flavor in those carbs, which include whole-grain bread, pasta, cereal, and brown rice, as well as other foods you might not expect, such as beans, fruit, vegetables, and low-fat dairy products. In Weeks 1, 2, and 5 of the Lean Plate Club Program you'll learn how to choose carbs wisely and how many carbs to eat daily. You'll even discover why enriched white carbs—a slice of warm French bread, a steaming bowl of white rice with Chinese food, or a serving of lasagna—can sometimes be smart choices.

Fat is not a four-letter word. Before there was a nutritional vendetta against carbohydrates, fat was considered the nutrient to avoid. Scientists have long shown that there are good fats and bad fats. The rest of us are just catching up with this concept. You likely know that saturated fat, cholesterol, and trans-fatty acids are fats to avoid. And you may even know about some of the healthy fats—olive oil and nuts, for example. But there's a whole lot more to learn about the good, the bad, and the oily. In Chapter Four, you'll find a brief nutritional primer that explains the many benefits of monounsaturated fats, such as olive or canola oils, why omega-3 fatty acids found in seafood are good for your heart, your brain, and your joints, and how to incorporate enough—but not too much—polyunsaturated fat, such as safflower oil. During Week 3 of the Lean Plate Club Program, you'll learn the secrets of trading the bad fats for the good.

Everyone needs a backup plan. Trust me, no matter how strong your motivation is today, no matter how dedicated you feel right now, sooner or later something will get in the way of your new, healthy efforts. Maybe your work will become more hectic. You'll switch jobs or find you have to travel more. Perhaps your family is about to expand. Or maybe a relative will suddenly need some extra care or attention. Nothing in life stays static. It's a matter of when—not if—life throws a wrench into your plans. One Lean Plate Club member was living with her husband and two young daughters in Vancouver, British Columbia, and making good progress to a healthier weight when her husband was transferred with just a week's notice to Toronto. She stayed behind with her two daughters to let them finish the school year before moving to Toronto. Despite the stress of moving her family, living briefly as a single parent, and relocating her law practice and filmmaking business to another city, she still managed to stay on track and has now lost more than 150 pounds. "It was a very stressful year," she said. "We moved three thousand miles, but I have made this my lifestyle. I think that is really key. I actually choose different foods to eat and have different portion sizes than I used to eat, and I eat a lot of vegetables. In fact, my favorite breakfast is now a veggie egg-substitute omelet with high-fiber toast and light margarine."

How you handle these kinds of life changes will make—or break—your long-term success. That's why in Week 8 you're going to learn how to develop and practice contingency plans for the days when life overtakes you. You'll also find sample menus and recipes, and learn how to plan at least a meal ahead to stay on track.

Support helps. Everybody needs encouragement, especially with weight loss. Studies show that it's a key element of long-term success. How much support you choose is up to you. In the pages ahead, you'll find effective ways to get the help and support you need from your family, friends, and colleagues as you move toward a healthier weight. You'll see how to enlist an exercise buddy to boost your odds of working out regularly. You'll learn how to draft help to avoid overeating at parties and where to find a sympathetic ear when the going gets tough. In addition to the dozens of secrets that you'll discover throughout this book to help you live like a thinner person, you'll soon have new tools to help you take stock of your body and will see how to set key achievable goals. Plus, you are now a member in good standing of the Lean Plate Club, which includes a large electronic community to provide support, motivation, and inspiration. You can participate in the weekly on-line Web chat, e-mail me personally anytime, solicit help online from other Lean Plate Club members, and subscribe to the weekly free e-mail Lean Plate Club newsletter, where you'll find lots more tips, the latest nutrition and exercise news, and ways to help boost physical activity or just keep your exercise regime fresh.

You have to make time—not find it—for healthy habits. "I just don't have time to do this" is a lament that I hear frequently. Truth is, you don't have time not to. We all get the same 168 hours each week. What differs is how we spend it.

Throughout the coming pages you'll see how Lean Plate Club members have learned to fit in meal planning, grocery shopping, healthy cooking, and regular workouts, whether they go to the gym, work out at home, or even exercise at their desks. Everyone is busy. As one Lean Plate Club member advised, "The trick for me is not to think about it! I go on autopilot when I get home from work. I have a routine where I check the weather on television as I change my clothes and get out the door to exercise. Don't overthink it. You owe it to yourself."

Healthy habits energize you. There's scientific evidence that eating smart and moving more enable you to feel sharper and more efficient. Plus, when you're well fueled, your blood sugar doesn't rise and fall sharply, which affects how hungry and tired you feel. When you're physically active, you improve blood flow and increase oxygen throughout your body—even if you don't reach peak aerobic levels during every workout. "I have the energy of a 20-year-old and the enthusiasm of a 10-year-old," says one 45-year-old Lean Plate Club member who now weighs 265 pounds but once tipped the scales at more than 400 pounds.

Mankato, Minn.: One good way to add spice to your daily walking is to check out books on tape from your local library. When I go for a walk I start listening to a book. The time goes so fast that sometimes I want to keep walking to hear more of the story. I always stick a couple of extra tapes in my pockets so I can continue when the first tape runs out.

The bottom line isn't just the number on the bathroom scale. Focus on the habits, and the pounds will fall into place. Weight loss doesn't always occur exactly at the rate you wish. In fact, it's not unusual for some people to lose more inches than pounds at first. "My clothes are looser and people tell me that I look thinner," one Lean Plate Club member noted. "But the scale hasn't moved yet." It's a well-documented phenomenon that scientists don't yet have an answer for, although many believe that it has to do with the body's readjustment of fat and lean body mass.

Others, especially those who are quite overweight or obese, may find that the scale moves steadily downward at first, then slows, and may even plateau before moving lower again. "When I was big, I could lose six pounds some weeks," said Arlene Rimer, who lost a total of 70 pounds before she hit her first plateau. It lasted four months.

The secret is that achieving a healthier weight is usually not

a straight downward path but a trend that can have plateaus and even a few brief upward spikes. In the pages ahead, you'll learn how to cope with these discouraging moments.

Or as a Lean Plate Club member who lost more than 100 pounds told me, "After years of trying various diets and setting lofty goals, I finally started out just saying that I needed to lose some weight. I didn't worry about the amount. I did the same thing week after week. For quite a while, the scale dropped a half pound or a pound every week. But then there were weeks when I did exactly the same things and the scale stayed steady. And some weeks when it even rose a little. I used to joke that the only difference seemed to be the way I parted my hair."

That's why it's fine to monitor the scale regularly but best not to get obsessed by it or to consider the numbers on the scale your only measure of success. In "Take Stock" on page 40 and in Chapter Three, you'll learn how to set reasonable goals, how to meet them, and how to measure your progress, not just your success. At more than 400 pounds, a Lean Plate Club member from northern Virginia found it difficult to walk just a block. When he added healthy eating habits, he lost weight steadily; then his weight stabilized for a couple of months. "In the old days, I would have gone back to my old habits," he said. "But it didn't bother me, because I feel so incredibly good." He's since shed more than 140 pounds and completely altered his daily habits. "It is taking time for me to reach my goal, but I look okay and I certainly feel okay, so that's all that matters," he said.

Give yourself permission to eat. Food is sustenance. That means it's okay to enjoy a healthy, balanced meal. And no, standing over the kitchen sink, eating directly out of the fridge, mindlessly consuming calories in front of the television, or chowing down in the car does not count. There was a reason that our ancestors stopped toiling, sat down, and ate at regular intervals throughout the day. Many Europeans continue this tradition, and their rates of overweight and obesity have risen more slowly than in the United States. Our nonstop noshing is endangering the age-old practice of eating regular, satisfying meals.

Somehow, in our fast-paced lives, we've lost sight of the fact that food is nourishment—not escape—and is meant to be savored. During the next eight weeks, you'll learn how to savor food. You'll see how Lean Plate Club members with lives as busy as yours have taken back control of their kitchens, dining rooms, and pantries. You can, too. In Week 8 of the Lean Plate Club Program, you'll practice mindful eating, learn how to tame food obsessions, and identify the trigger foods that can fuel your overeating.

Nothing is off-limits. Make foods forbidden, especially any favorite foods, and it's likely that you'll want them even more. So unless you break out in hives or are otherwise allergic to a particular food, there are no foods to avoid with the Lean Plate Club. But that doesn't give you license to consume unlimited amounts of your favorite high-calorie fare. "Everything in moderation" is one of the mottoes of the Lean Plate Club.

In the weeks ahead you'll learn how to put that motto into practice, as did this member from Coral Springs, Florida: "I allow myself one small treat each day. I really love chocolate, so I look forward to treating myself to a small amount, such as half a brownie (and looking forward to the other half tomorrow!) or a snack-size candy bar, or sharing a dessert at a restaurant. If I know I'm going to eat out, I don't have a treat during the day so that I can look forward to dessert. When faced with a number of tempting choices, I pick the one that I feel I will enjoy the most or don't otherwise have the opportunity to taste very often. I've been using this strategy for about ten years now, and I never feel like I'm missing out on anything."

It's never too late to work toward a healthier weight. It doesn't matter whether you're 18 or 81. It doesn't matter if you're just a bit overweight or morbidly obese. Eating smart and moving more help people of all ages, shapes, and fitness levels feel better, and there's solid scientific evidence of important health benefits from doing so. The federally funded Diabetes Prevention Trial showed that people on the cusp of developing diabetes who lost only 7 percent of their body weight lowered their risk of developing diabetes by nearly 60 percent. For a 200-pound person, that is about 14 pounds. Same goes for exercise. It's never too late to reap the health benefits. Studies at Tufts University show that even 90-year-old nursing-home residents benefit from weight training by strengthening their muscles. Imagine what it can do for you.

You need to believe you can succeed. Thinking is as important as eating and exercise when it comes to weight loss. Research shows that the best predictor of success is something called self-efficacy—how confident you are that you can achieve your goals. Even if you've tried and failed numerous times before, you're going to discover proven ways to boost your belief that you can reach a healthier weight, as did a Lean Plate Club member from Sedona, Arizona, who also found a new calling as a volunteer firefighter in the process. "I just wanted to say thanks for your column. It, along with the many resources mentioned in the Web chat and motivation from some of my friends and Lean Plate Club members, has kept me on the path to healthy living these past couple of years. First I started by getting back into the sport I love: soccer. Then worked up to running a marathon. Now, I finally feel fit enough—and, most important, confident enough—to pursue something that I had put off for a long time: being a firefighter. I passed all the initial tests last week and start firefighter/emergency medical training classes next month, paid for by the local fire district. I just wanted to say thanks to you and the other members of the Lean Plate Club for the part they played in my progress!"

Keep it fresh. The trick for long-term weight-loss success is to find the right balance between healthy habits—which, by their very nature, are repetitive—and boredom that is likely to sabotage your efforts. The daily jogs that at first feel invigorating could seem monotonous in six months. The hearty soups that taste inviting and warm today may seem tired and unappealing a few months from now. Doing the same old thing can get routine very fast. You'll see how to keep your new healthy habits fresh and vital so that you don't become bored or burned out. Discovering water aerobics helped one Lean Plate Club member from Washington, D.C., turn a corner to healthy habits. "About a year and a half ago I was 100 pounds overweight. I was afraid to exercise. Finally, I started doing water aerobics one or two times a week. It was the best thing that ever happened to me. It was so simple to do and the stress was taken away from my joints. The thing that struck me most is that once I started moving, the weight started to come off. It was small at first, but with the combination of the Lean Plate Club and small amounts of regular exercise, I've shed most of the 100 pounds I needed to lose."

Practice, practice, practice. The eight-week Lean Plate Club Program puts you well on your way toward achieving a healthier weight. But that's just the beginning. Behavioral research shows that it takes at least weeks, often months and even years, for some new habits to take hold. So you'll learn how to use those initial eight weeks as a springboard for long-term success. "Three and a half years ago, I was in such bad shape physically that merely sweeping off my front porch left me breathless," said a Lean Plate Club member from Gaithersburg, Maryland, who has lost 80 pounds and kept it off for several years. "I started exercising slowly and graduated from a CardioGlide to a bicycle. I could bike only four miles at first and I got nauseated, but I stuck with it. Today, I can ride 50 to 60 miles at a time and am in as good a shape as when I was in my twenties."

Satisfaction leads to success. Unless you feel full and satisfied, odds are you won't stick with any new eating regimen for long. Few people can tolerate feeling chronically hungry and deprived. The Lean Plate Club shows you how to feel full on fewer calories, based on clinically proven findings from well-respected scientists at leading universities. You'll learn the importance of regular meals and portion control, and the value of consuming high-volume foods that fill you up with fewer calories. Plus, you'll discover the most effective ways to work out without fueling your appetite, as well as what to eat before and after exercising to optimize both endurance and fat burning.

Know how to recover from slips so that they don't become slides into failure. Everybody has a bad day. Or a bad week. Or even a bad month. Learning how to get back on track after nutritional mischief and bouts of inactivity is essential for long-term success. In the weeks ahead, you'll learn how to sidestep guilt trips and coach yourself back to healthy habits, as does this Lean Plate Club member who has successfully maintained a 20-pound weight loss for more than two years: "I find that when I look good, I take better care of myself. Also, I make it a hard-and-fast rule: no second trips to those killer buffets. And if I fall off the wagon, I'm sure to climb right back on. That has been the most important lesson for me. Even if I overindulge on a trip or at a party, I know that each day comes with an opportunity to begin anew."

Reward yourself. Most people never give themselves even a pat on the back for achieving a healthier weight. When you set a goal, whether small or large, you'll also learn the importance of rewarding yourself for meeting that goal. It can be as simple as soaking in a candlelit bubble bath or downloading a tune that you've wanted for your iPod, or as fancy as splurging on a facial, massage, or pedicure. Each week, you'll be reminded to provide a new reward to reinforce your efforts.

Arlington, Va.: Hi, Sally—Just wanted to report that I've lost five pounds in the month and a half that I've been following along with the LPC. I was in pretty good shape before, but I've cleaned up my diet (more whole grains, fruits, and veggies, less meat and cheese) and have increased my activity level so that I'm getting a solid work-out at least five days a week. Now that the weather has gotten nice, I've been riding my bike to and from work one or two days a week (14 miles round-trip). Thanks for all the suggestions. Keep them coming.

Crave activity. Thirty-eight percent of American adults are so sedentary that they engage in *no activity* during leisure hours. None. Zip. Nada. That missed opportunity undermines efforts at weight loss. During the next eight weeks, you'll learn how to boost your daily physical activity level whether you're a couch potato, a dedicated gym rat, or something in between. Let's face it, modern conveniences are engineering activity out of our lives, so even if you do go to the gym for an hour daily, odds are that you're still inactive for the other 23 hours each day.

You don't need to limit yourself to jogging, weight training, or playing popular sports such as tennis or golf. A number of Lean Plate Club members are getting fit with less traditional methods, from the Japanese martial art aikido to the fast-moving Argentinean tango. "I started studying belly dancing a couple of years ago," one Lean Plate Club member reported, "and have been delighted with how well it's kept me interested and motivated after all those years that I hated exercise! I cannot recommend it highly enough. It's an excellent low-impact workout, great for flexibility and cardiovascular fitness, and works for women of all shapes and sizes. Even men!"

The only failure is in no longer trying. Studies show that it often takes at least a half-dozen attempts to succeed long term at weight loss, a fact that seems to be missing from most diet books and weight-loss programs. In a few pages, you'll have a chance to review your weight-loss history, gauge how ready you are to begin to instill healthy eating and physical activity habits, and take stock of where your body stands today. View this as an opportunity, since even if you're a veteran yo-yo dieter, behavioral research shows that each time you've shed weight—despite regaining it—you've still learned something important about what works and doesn't work for you. Now you're ready to put it all together. Turn the page and *Secrets of the Lean Plate Club* will begin to show you how.

Two

ARE YOU READY TO ACHIEVE A HEALTHIER WEIGHT?

Whether this is your first attempt at weight loss or your tenth or your hundredth, it's important to take stock of your current weight and to examine how and why your weight has changed through the years. You will likely discover patterns that you never recognized before.

Your first option is to start right here with these four steps. But if you'd prefer, you can also jump ahead to Week 1 of the Lean Plate Club Program and begin right away. (The only thing you'll need to do is to calculate your daily calorie goal. Find out how to do that in Chapter Three.)

Your second option is to take these self-tests, which are designed to help you do a little introspection and ask a few questions of yourself to help establish your goals. These tests are brief. You can do them at one sitting or spread them out over a day or two. The choice, like everything else in this book, is up to you. The one thing that writing the Lean Plate Club column and hosting the Web chat has taught me over the past five years is this: You're the best judge of what works well for you.

Step 1. Examine your weight history. Have you battled weight problems since childhood, or added pounds as an adult? Did your waistline expand after a pregnancy or because of the stress of a difficult job, a move to a new city, a divorce, retirement, or something else? Are you a yo-yo dieter? The questions and chart on pages 24 to 27 will help you take a closer look at your weight problems.

Step 2. Use the Weight Loss Readiness Test on page 29 to help assess your to ability to embark on habit changes during the eight-week Lean Plate Club Program.

Step 3. Check out your body. You will need a soft tape measure and a bathroom scale, plus a small notebook, journal, PDA, or other way to record measurements.

Step 4. Take the PAR-Q test for exercise. Depending on your results, check with your physician or health-care provider before becoming more physically active.

WHY ARE WE GETTING FATTER?
Average calories consumed daily in the U.S.

Bottom line: + 300 calories a day is enough to pile on 30 pounds per year.

1985	2,200
2000	2,500

SOURCES: U.S. Department of Agriculture; National Center for Health Statistics

---

STEP 1. YOUR WEIGHT HISTORY

Please list your weight beginning in your teens until the present. Then photocopy the chart on pages 24 and 25 and graph your weight through the years. It takes about five minutes to do the chart.

"Jane's" experience is typical of many. She put on the "freshman 15" during her first year at college, thanks to extra helpings at the cafeteria, indulging in beer and pizza on weekends, and cutting back on the volleyball and basketball that she'd played competitively in high school. She dropped ten pounds when she moved to an off-campus apartment, started cooking healthier meals for herself and her roommates, and began regular workouts at the college gym. She and one of her roommates also jogged together three to four times per week. Jane managed to maintain these habits and keep her weight steady until graduation, but on her first job, she spent most of her time at a desk. She couldn't afford a gym membership and didn't live close enough to walk to work.

At her office, a coworker who loved to bake brought in a constant supply of high-calorie tempting treats. Jane quickly gained five pounds and began a familiar pattern. Each Monday, she'd vow to lose weight. She tried a variety of restrictive diets. By Friday, she felt she had earned the right to splurge on the weekends with her friends.

Like many, Jane saw her "diet" as all or none. When she was good—as she was during the week—she was very, very good and almost became too restrained with her eating. But when she was "bad," as she described it, she went overboard.

On Monday, she felt guilty, stepped on the bathroom scale, and found she had regained the weight lost the week before. Back she went on another restrictive diet, starting a vicious cycle. Over the next several years, she tried all kinds of weight-loss regimens with varying degrees of success and set up a chronic pattern of yo-yo dieting, each time gradually regaining the weight lost, plus a couple more pounds.

Before her wedding, Jane worked very hard to shed about 15 pounds. She and her husband loved to cook and often ate out with friends. So by the time they celebrated their first wedding anniversary, Jane had regained all 15 pounds she'd lost before getting married. She managed to maintain her weight for two more years until she became pregnant. Then she gained 50 pounds, about twice what her obstetrician recommended.

After her daughter was born, Jane bought a treadmill, ate three regular meals daily, and took off about 20 pregnancy-related pounds. She maintained that weight until she became pregnant two years later with her second child and gained another 30 pounds. Caring for two young children and working part-time left little time for meal planning, cooking, or exercise. Dinner for Jane and her husband was often fast-food takeout, loaded with calories and fat. Her weight continued to climb. Later, when Jane returned to work full-time and had a lengthy commute, more pounds crept on. Jane realized that she couldn't put off addressing her out-of-control weight any longer.

By reviewing her body weight and charting it over the years, Jane had an epiphany: Her attempts of very restrictive eating only resulted in yo-yo dieting. She also figured out that she had been most successful at weight control when she found ways to exercise daily and eat regular, healthy meals. At those times, she didn't feel ravenous or out of control and was less apt to gorge on what-

---

How many calories it takes to lose

1 pound = 3,500
2 pounds = 7,000
5 pounds = 17,500
10 pounds = 35,000
15 pounds = 52,500
20 pounds = 70,000
25 pounds = 87,500
30 pounds = 105,000
35 pounds = 122,500
40 pounds = 140,000
45 pounds = 157,500
50 pounds = 175,000
75 pounds = 262,500
100 pounds = 350,000

---

ever tempting food happened to be around. She also noticed that when she exercised with a friend, as she had done in college, she was much more likely to stick with her workout plans.

James had a different experience. When he charted his weight, he realized that his weight battles began well after college. Most of his extra pounds piled on during study for the bar exam and the seven years he spent working 70-hour weeks at his firm. That's when James subsisted on greasy take-out food and gave up his noon basketball game at the Y and virtually all other physical activity. No wonder he put on 30 pounds.

As James charted his weight, he recalled that he successfully trimmed about ten pounds before his wedding. But he regained weight during his wife's pregnancy—sympathy pounds—and even more after their son was born. The couple spent what little free time they had sitting in front of the television and, invariably, eating. James got a wake-up call when he was diagnosed with elevated blood cholesterol levels and high blood pressure.

He joined a gym, began taking two prescription medications to lower his cholesterol and blood pressure, and changed his diet. A little. But the birth of a second child meant that he spent what little free time he had at home—and no time at the gym or working out. His weight began to rise again, reaching an all-time high. James's doctor warned that he was flirting with some very serious health problems unless he took action.

In reviewing his weight history and chart, James realized that he was most successful in controlling his weight when he stayed very physically active, avoided nonstop stress snacking, and drank less alcohol.

Now, take a look at your weight history. What patterns do you see? Where have you had success? What's led to your weight gain or weight cycling? What trajectory are you on unless you take steps now to reach a healthier weight?

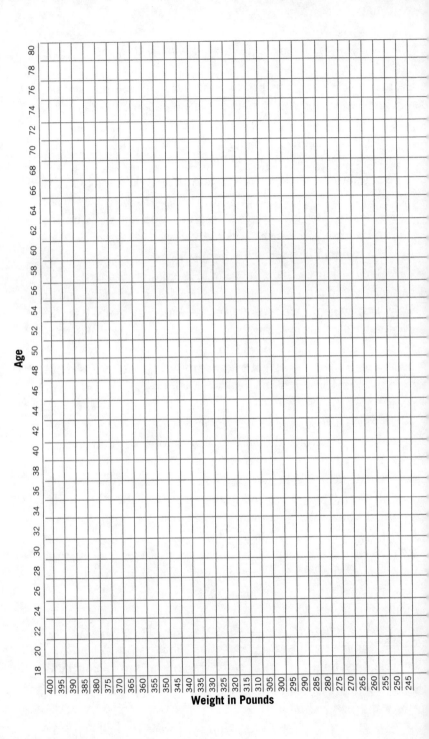

Age

Weight in Pounds

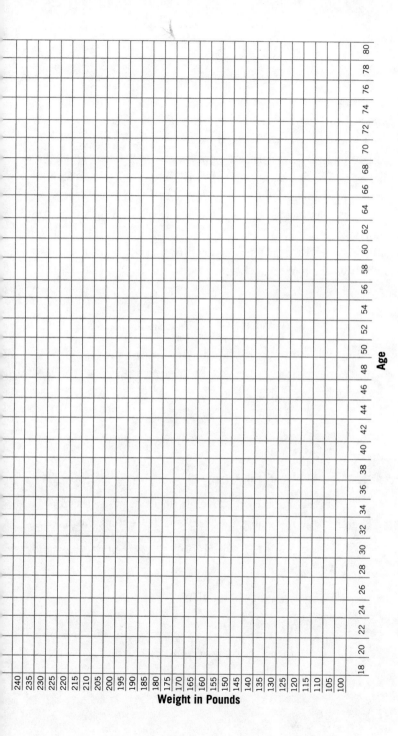

Weight in Pounds

240 235 230 225 220 215 210 205 200 195 190 185 180 175 170 165 160 155 150 145 140 135 130 125 120 115 110 105 100

18 20 22 24 26 28 30 32 34 36 38 40 42 44 46 48 50 52 54 56 58 60 62 64 66 68 70 72 74 76 78 80

Age

The Weight Loss Redux questionnaire provided below will also help you to get a better handle on your weight history and weight-loss patterns of success and failure. Use the answers to help you assess what's worked—and what hasn't—in past weight-loss attempts. Before setting new goals, analyze how quickly you have lost weight in the past, when you were most successful at trimming pounds, and what prompted their return. Try to reflect on what was happening in your life as your weight fluctuated. Marriage? Pregnancy? Divorce? Job change? A health problem for a loved one? Relocation? The declining health or death of a parent? If you're like most people, you will see patterns emerge.

WEIGHT LOSS REDUX

How many times have you tried to lose weight? _____

How many times have you been successful at reaching your goal weight? _____

What methods have you used to lose weight?

- ____ Ate less

- ____ Got more physical activity

- ____ Joined a commercial weight-loss program (Weight Watchers, Jenny Craig, LA Weight Loss Centers, etc.)

- ____ Joined a self-help group (TOPS, Overeaters Anonymous, Food Addicts)

- ____ Followed a diet-book plan

- ____ Used meal replacements

- ____ Tried nonprescription weight-loss medication

- ____ Took weight-loss drugs prescribed by a physician

- ____ Had bariatric surgery (gastric bypass, stomach stapling)

- ____ Fasting

- ____ Jaw wiring

What approach worked best? _____

List the reasons that you succeeded. (For example, maybe a friend, colleague, or family member participated with you.)

_____

_____

_____

_____

_____

How long were you successful at maintaining your weight loss? _____

Take a few minutes to consider your answers:

- **What do you see that accounts for your past success?** Did you have more time to spend on cooking or meal planning? Did you have a regular time to work out? Was physical activity more convenient? Perhaps you had an easier commute or a shorter workday. Maybe you belonged to a gym, had a standing weekly doubles tennis game, or got into the habit of pedaling your stationary bike every morning while you read the paper.

- **How about your slips?** Did they occur suddenly, such as when you found yourself under stress or very tired? Did a slip happen when you followed a very rigid or restrictive diet? Or perhaps your slips were triggered by skipping meals and then feeling ravenous. Did your detours from healthy habits occur gradually—you know, an extra helping now and then at dinner, or a regular afternoon soft drink combined with less and less exercise? Or is nonstop overeating your problem, particularly at night? Examine your slips closely to find important clues to the triggers that send you in the wrong direction. Then consider strategies that could help prevent them in the future. (You'll find more help in Chapter Fourteen.)

- **What about your weight-loss goals?** Were they realistic? Did you overestimate, underestimate, or correctly calculate what you could lose each week? Did you ever meet your goal?

- **How did you approach maintaining your weight loss?** Did you make any special plans, or just hope that "things would take care of themselves"? Research clearly shows that long-term weight maintenance takes focus and commitment. But the good news is that it also gets easier with time.

Tired of Counting Pounds?

Consider tracking percent body fat, made possible by a number of devices that look just like a standard bathroom scale. The difference is that they use a tiny electric current, also known as bioimpedance, to estimate your percent body fat. Don't worry: The current is so tiny that you can't feel it.

Combination scale and fat counters start at about $25 and go up to more than $1,000. They are available at bed and bath shops, department stores, and on the Web. Some will even calculate how many calories you need to maintain or lose weight.

For about $15, you can buy calipers to measure your percent body fat at home. Fancier calipers with digital readings can run as much as $150. None of these devices are as accurate as bioelectrical impedance or underwater testing—the way that researchers measure body fat.

STEP 2. WEIGHT LOSS READINESS TEST II

Kelly Brownell, Ph.D., director of the Yale Center for Eating and Weight Disorders, developed this psychological tool with David L. Hager, Ph.D., and Beth Leermakers, Ph.D., to test your readiness to shed pounds. The following questions will help you assess your motivation, expectations, confidence, perceptions of hunger, and various other things to gauge your chance of success.

Answer the questions below to see how well your attitudes and current behaviors equip you for a weight-loss program. For each question, circle the number that best describes your attitude, then write the number of your answer next to each question. As you complete each of the six categories, add the number of your answers and compare them with the scoring guide at the end of this test.

Category 1: Motivation

1. Compared to previous attempts, how motivated are you to lose weight at this time?
  0   Not at all motivated
  1   Slightly motivated
  2   Somewhat motivated
  3   Quite motivated
  4   Extremely motivated

2. Compared to previous attempts, how motivated are you to change your eating habits this time?
  0   Not at all motivated
  1   Slightly motivated
  2   Somewhat motivated
  3   Quite motivated
  4   Extremely motivated

3. Compared to previous attempts, how motivated are you to increase your physical activity this time?

0   Not at all motivated
1   Slightly motivated
2   Somewhat motivated
3   Quite motivated
4   Extremely motivated

4. How motivated are you to stay committed to a weight-loss program for the time it will take to reach your weight-loss goal?

0   Not at all motivated
1   Slightly motivated
2   Somewhat motivated
3   Quite motivated
4   Extremely motivated

5. How motivated are you to try new strategies/techniques for changing your eating, exercise, and other behaviors?

0   Not at all motivated
1   Slightly motivated
2   Somewhat motivated
3   Quite motivated
4   Extremely motivated

Category 1 Motivation total score _____

Category 2: Expectations

6. Think honestly about how much weight you hope to lose and how quickly you hope to lose it. Figuring a weight loss of one to two pounds per week, how realistic is your expectation?

0 Very unrealistic
1 Somewhat unrealistic
2 Moderately unrealistic
3 Somewhat realistic
4 Very realistic

7. How satisfied would you be if you achieved a 10 percent weight loss? (For example, if you weigh 200 pounds, that works out to 20 pounds.)
0 Not at all satisfied
1 Slightly satisfied
2 Somewhat satisfied
3 Quite satisfied
4 Extremely satisfied

8. If you achieved a 10 percent weight loss that significantly improved your health, how satisfied would you be?
0 Not at all satisfied
1 Slightly satisfied
2 Somewhat satisfied
3 Quite satisfied
4 Extremely satisfied

9. If you achieved a 10 percent weight loss that significantly improved your quality of life, how satisfied would you be?
0 Not at all satisfied
1 Slightly satisfied
2 Somewhat satisfied
3 Quite satisfied
4 Extremely satisfied

Category 2 Expectations total score _____

Category 3: Confidence

When answering questions 10 through 17, consider all outside factors at this time in your life (the stress you're feeling at work and/or home, your obligations, etc.).

10. People who want to achieve long-term weight control need to spend time every day trying to change their eating, exercise, and thinking habits. You probably know the time and commitment necessary for you to be successful. How confident are you that you can devote this amount of effort, both now and over the next few months?

  0   Not at all confident
  1   Slightly confident
  2   Somewhat confident
  3   Quite confident
  4   Extremely confident

11. How confident are you that you will be able to attend program meetings regularly or, if you are not in a formal program, follow your own program regularly?

  0   Not at all confident
  1   Slightly confident
  2   Somewhat confident
  3   Quite confident
  4   Extremely confident

12. How confident are you that you will be able to record everything you eat and drink and your exercise most days of the week?

  0   Not at all confident
  1   Slightly confident
  2   Somewhat confident

3   Quite confident
4   Extremely confident

13. How confident are you that you will be able to change your eating habits?
0   Not at all confident
1   Slightly confident
2   Somewhat confident
3   Quite confident
4   Extremely confident

14. How confident are you that you will be able to work regular physical activity into your daily schedule?
0   Not at all confident
1   Slightly confident
2   Somewhat confident
3   Quite confident
4   Extremely confident

15. How confident are you that you will be able to exercise at least five days per week, most weeks?
0   Not at all confident
1   Slightly confident
2   Somewhat confident
3   Quite confident
4   Extremely confident

16. How confident are you that you will be able to maintain your healthy eating habits for one year or longer?
0   Not at all confident
1   Slightly confident
2   Somewhat confident

3   Quite confident
4   Extremely confident

17. How confident are you that you will be able to continue exercising regularly (at least five days per week) for one year or longer?

0   Not at all confident
1   Slightly confident
2   Somewhat confident
3   Quite confident
4   Extremely confident

Category 3 Confidence total score _____

Category 4: Hunger and Eating Cues

18. When food comes up in conversation or in something you read, do you want to eat even if you are not hungry?

0   Never
1   Rarely
2   Occasionally
3   Frequently
4   Always

19. How often do you eat because of physical hunger?

0   Always
1   Frequently
2   Occasionally
3   Rarely
4   Never

20. Do you have trouble controlling your eating when your favorite foods are around the house?

0   Never
1   Rarely
2   Occasionally
3   Frequently
4   Always

Category 4 Hunger and Eating Cues total score _____

Category 5: Binge Eating and Purging

21. Aside from holiday feasts, have you ever eaten a large amount of food rapidly and felt afterward that this eating incident was excessive and out of control?

2   Yes
0   No

22. If you answered yes to question 21, above, how often have you engaged in this behavior during the last year?

0   Less than once a month
1   About once a month
2   A few times a month
3   About once a week
4   About three times a week
5   Daily

23. Have you ever purged (used laxatives, diuretics, or induced vomiting) to control your weight?

3   Yes
0   No

24. If you answered yes to question 23, how often have you engaged in this behavior during the last year?

0   Less than once a month
1   About once a month
2   A few times a month
3   About once a week
4   About three times a week
5   Daily

Category 5 Binge Eating and Purging total score _____

Category 6: Emotional Eating

25. Do you eat more than you would like to when you have negative feelings, such as anxiety, depression, anger, or loneliness?

0   Never
1   Rarely
2   Occasionally
3   Frequently
4   Always

26. Do you have trouble controlling your eating when you have positive feelings—do you celebrate feeling good by eating?

0   Never
1   Rarely
2   Occasionally
3   Frequently
4   Always

27. When you have unpleasant interactions with others in your life, or after a difficult day at work, do you eat more than you would like?

0   Never
1   Rarely
2   Occasionally
3   Frequently
4   Always

Category 6 Emotional Eating total score _____

SCORING

Category 1: Motivation

If you scored

0–6:   This may not be a good time for you to start a weight-loss program. Inadequate motivation could block your progress. Think about the things that contribute to this, and consider changing them before undertaking a weight-loss program. *(This is a great time, however, to hold the line on further weight gain. Find additional information and help in Chapter Three.)*

7–14:   You may be close to being ready to begin a weight-loss program but should think about ways to increase your motivation before you begin. *(While you ponder that, do maintain your weight and consider setting a start date within the next week or two to begin lose weight.)*

15–20:   The path is clear with respect to your motivation.

Category 2: Expectations

If you scored

0–5:   Your expectations for weight loss are unrealistic. If you do not achieve your weight-loss goals, you will probably be very disappointed. Think about your reasons for losing weight and try to set more realistic goals.

6–11:   Your expectations may be a bit high. Try to focus on other reasons for changing your eating and exercise behavior besides just the numbers on the scale.

12–16:   Your expectations are right on target.

Category 3: Confidence

If you scored

0–12:   This may not be a good time for you to start a weight-loss program. You may want to wait until you feel more confident in your ability to change your behavior. *(You could, however, still hold the line on further weight gain. See Chapter 3 for more information.)*

13–23:   You may be close to being ready to begin a weight-loss program but should think about ways to boost your confidence before you begin.

24–32:   Your confidence in your ability to change your behavior is strong.

Category 4: Hunger and Eating Cues

If you scored

0–3:   You might occasionally eat more than you would like, but it does not appear to be a result of high responsiveness to external cues. Controlling the attitudes that make you eat may be especially helpful.

4–6:   You may have a moderate tendency to eat just because food is available. Weight loss may be easier for you if you try to resist external cues, and eat only when you are physically hungry. (*See Chapter Twelve for more on taming mindless eating.*)

7–12:   Some or most of your eating may be in response to thinking about food or exposing yourself to temptations to eat. Think of ways to minimize your exposure to temptations— and learn more in Chapter Twelve—so that you eat only in response to physical hunger.

Category 5: Binge Eating and Purging

If you scored

0–2:   It appears that binge eating and purging are not problems for you.

3–5:   Pay attention to these eating patterns. If they interfere with your life or concern you, see a professional. Definitely see a professional if they get worse.

6–15:   Be aware of potentially having a serious eating problem, particularly if your score is high in this range and the problems are current. In this case, see a counselor experienced in evaluating and treating eating disorders.

Category 6: Emotional Eating

If you scored

0–5:   You do not appear to let your emotions affect your eating.

6–8:   You sometimes eat in response to emotional highs and lows. Monitor this behavior to learn when and why it occurs, and be prepared to find alternative activities.

9–12:   Emotional ups and downs can stimulate your eating. Try to deal with the feelings that trigger the eating and find other ways to express them.

Reproduced with permission. All rights reserved. Brownell, K. D., D. L. Hager, E. Leermakers. The Weight Loss Readiness Test II—2004. Version 5.4. Dallas, Tex.: American Health Publishing Company. All rights reserved. For ordering information call toll-free 1-888-LEARN-41 or visit www.TheLifeStyleCompany.com.

STEP 3. TAKE STOCK

Maybe you avoid mirrors. Or you haven't weighed yourself since New Year's Day five years ago. It can be sobering—even painful to your psyche—to get on a bathroom scale, but you need to do it. Unless you know the score, you can't possibly begin to track your progress. Think of it in financial terms: You wouldn't buy a house, plan a wedding, or take a vacation without first knowing the balance in your bank account.

Can't fit on your bathroom scale at home? You aren't the first to face that problem. See if you can get weighed at a doctor's office, clinic, or hospital.

Or do what physician Nick Yphantides did. Before quitting his job and embarking on a very public, major yearlong effort, which he chronicled in *My Big Fat Greek Diet,* Yphantides placed two identical scales on his living room floor. He put one foot on each scale and, with his physician brother as a witness, added up the total: a whopping 467 pounds.

Imperfect? Perhaps, but it gave him a ballpark body weight measurement and started Yphantides on a successful life change. Through an unusual regimen that wouldn't be for everyone, he lost 257 pounds in a year—without surgery—and still maintains a healthy weight.

So summon up your courage to climb on the scale, preferably in the morning as soon as you wake up. It's a good idea to weigh yourself au naturel just after rising and after urinating. Place your bathroom scale on a hard, flat surface. If that requires moving the scale from where it usually sits, mark the spot with some tape, so you can place it there again and obtain a consistent reading in the days and weeks to come.

If you use a combination scale/bioelectrical impedance device to measure your body fat, ask how it is calibrated. Most use software designed for the population where they are sold. The devices sold in the United States and Europe are generally calibrated to a Caucasian body type, and may be less accurate for those of other racial heritages.

The point is to find the most accurate measurement possible. You may also want to use a combination scale and body fat percentage device. These tools run about $25 to $1,000 and send a tiny electric current (you can't feel it, I promise) throughout your body to measure your percentage of body fat. These devices are not as accurate as the more expensive underwater body fat testing: the Dual Energy X-ray Absorptiometery (DEXA) test, which usually is done in a hospital and requires a very tiny exposure to radiation; or the Bod Pod, which uses sensors in a podlike device to determine percentage of body fat (www.bodpod.com). Record your weight and the date (more about that later). For men, optimal body fat ranges are 10 to 15 percent, 18 to 23 percent is average, 25 percent or more is obese. For women, 17 to 22 percent is considered optimal, 25 to 29 percent is average, and 35 percent or higher is obese.

While you're at it, this is also a good time to take a closer look at yourself in a full-length mirror. If you're like many people, you may feel a little squeamish or shy about giving yourself a once-over, particularly if you feel overweight and out of shape. Go ahead, take a look. Yes, that means turning a full 360 degrees. It's the only way to learn what you've got to work with. Truth is, you may be surprised at what you find, and it's a great way to reconnect with your body. People who become overweight often have one of two reactions to their bodies: They deny to themselves how much weight they've gained and do everything—including not looking in mirrors—to avoid any reminders, or they imagine the extra pounds to be far worse than they really are.

So come on, face your body. No matter what your weight, everybody has at least one good body part, even if it's a shapely ankle, a slender wrist, great shoulders, or the hint of a waist that could soon be a lot smaller. The importance of looking closely at your body goes far beyond vanity. Research suggests that overweight people who have better body images than their counterparts are more likely to be successful at making healthy eating and exercise changes. So find something you like about your body and build from there.

What about the other body parts that need work? Use them to your advantage. Have a jiggly middle? Remember that the next time you consider skipping a brisk walk or other aerobic activity. Flabby arms? That could be a good motivator to do some upper-body weight training and push-ups several times weekly. Do you have thunder thighs that block light between your legs? Use that for inspiration the next time you do lower-body resistance training, stair climbing, ballroom dancing, or step aerobics, since all these activities help sculpt your lower body—along with helping you achieve a healthier weight.

Finally, don a bathing suit or skintight shorts and top or a leotard. Ask a friend or family member to take your picture. Still too self-conscious? Then snap one of yourself in the full-length mirror. Put this "before" photo in a private place. No need to share it with anyone. Use it both for motivation and as a reminder in the weeks ahead of how much you have accomplished.

Body Mass Index (BMI)

With your current body weight in hand, turn to the body mass index calculator on pages 46 and 47 to find your BMI.

A quick word about the BMI. It's a tool that is based on height and weight and is routinely used to determine whether you are overweight, obese, or at risk for weight-related complications, such as type 2 diabetes, high blood pressure, or heart disease.

The advantage of the BMI is that it's simple to use and requires only one chart for men and women. A BMI of less than 18.5 is considered underweight. A healthy range is 18.5 to 24.9; 25 to 29.9 is overweight; greater than 30 is obese; higher than 40 is considered morbidly obese.

Like all tools, the BMI has shortcomings. It can overestimate weight-related health risks in muscular athletes with a BMI of 25 to 30. It is also less accurate in calculating risk for the elderly, who lose muscle mass as they age. Often, the BMI shows them as being at a healthy weight, when they may have a higher percentage of body fat than younger people.

Growing evidence also suggests that the BMI falls short for some non-Caucasian racial groups, giving them a false sense of security. In 2000, the World Health Organization's Pacific Group advised lowering the threshold for what is considered overweight in Asian populations to a BMI of 23 and making a BMI of 25 the beginning level for obesity, since health problems may emerge at BMI levels that are otherwise considered healthy.

Those of African and Polynesian descent tend to have a higher amount of lean muscle mass than Asians and Caucasians. So a BMI reading alone may cause them unnecessary worry. Some scientists believe that a BMI of 26 should be the threshold for what is considered overweight in these groups and a BMI of 32 the beginning of obesity. Whether specific BMI levels for other racial groups should also be set, such as for Hispanics or Native Americans, is still under discussion. In the Middle East, the number of adults who are overweight or obese has surged in the last 20 years, posing a health problem even greater than that in the United States.

PROPOSED RACIAL DIFFERENCES IN BODY MASS INDEX

	Overweight	Obese
Aboriginal including native tribes of Australia and New Zealand	23	25
African including African Americans	26	32
American and European	25	30
Asian Cambodia, China, India, Indonesia, Japan, Korea, North Korea, Singapore, Thailand, Vietnam, and other Asian countries	23	25
Hispanic	25	30
Middle Eastern	25	30
Native American	25	30
Polynesian including other South Pacific islands	26	32

SOURCES: World Health Organization; National Institutes of Health

So why use the BMI at all? Because experts say that it's still a good starting point to gauge your weight-related health risks and get a rough idea of whether you're moving toward the overweight or obese categories. If you combine BMI with your waist size, the accuracy for assessing risk appears much improved. So check your BMI on pages 46 and 47 and then get your tape measure ready to measure your waistline.

BODY MASS INDEX

Find your height in the left-hand column. Find your weight. The number at the top of the column is your body mass index.

BMI	19	20	21	22	23	24	25	26	27	28	29	30	31	32	33	34	35
Height (inches)	Body weight (pounds)																
58	91	96	100	105	110	115	119	124	129	134	138	143	148	153	158	162	167
59	94	99	104	109	114	119	124	128	133	138	143	148	153	158	163	168	173
60	97	102	107	112	118	123	128	133	138	143	148	153	158	163	168	174	179
61	100	106	111	116	122	127	132	137	143	148	153	158	164	169	174	180	185
62	104	109	115	120	126	131	136	142	147	153	158	164	169	175	180	186	191
63	107	113	118	124	130	135	141	146	152	158	163	169	175	180	186	191	197
64	110	116	122	128	134	140	145	151	157	163	169	174	180	186	192	197	204
65	114	120	126	132	138	144	150	156	162	168	174	180	186	192	198	204	210
66	118	124	130	136	142	148	155	161	167	173	179	186	192	198	204	210	216
67	121	127	134	140	146	153	159	166	172	178	185	191	198	204	211	217	223
68	125	131	138	144	151	158	164	171	177	184	190	197	203	210	216	223	230
69	128	135	142	149	155	162	169	176	182	189	196	203	209	216	223	230	236
70	132	139	146	153	160	167	174	181	188	195	202	209	216	222	229	236	243
71	136	143	150	157	165	172	179	186	193	200	208	215	222	229	236	243	250
72	140	147	154	162	169	177	184	191	199	206	213	221	228	235	242	250	258
73	144	151	159	166	174	182	189	197	204	212	219	227	235	242	250	257	265
74	148	155	163	171	179	186	194	202	210	218	225	233	241	249	256	264	272
75	152	160	168	176	184	192	200	208	216	224	232	240	248	256	264	272	279
76	156	164	172	180	189	197	205	213	221	230	238	246	254	263	271	279	287

BMI	36	37	38	39	40	41	42	43	44	45	46	47	48	49	50	51	52	53	54
Height (inches)	Body weight (pounds)																		
58	172	177	181	186	191	196	201	205	210	215	220	224	229	234	239	244	248	253	258
59	178	183	188	193	198	203	208	212	217	222	227	232	237	242	247	252	257	262	267
60	184	189	194	199	204	209	215	220	225	230	235	240	245	250	255	261	266	271	276
61	190	195	201	206	211	217	222	227	232	238	243	248	254	259	264	269	275	280	285
62	196	202	207	213	218	224	229	235	240	246	251	256	262	267	273	278	284	289	295
63	203	208	214	220	225	231	237	242	248	254	259	265	270	276	282	287	293	299	304
64	209	215	221	227	232	238	244	250	256	262	267	273	279	285	291	296	302	308	314
65	216	222	228	234	240	246	252	258	264	270	276	282	288	294	300	306	312	318	324
66	223	229	235	241	247	253	260	266	272	278	284	291	297	303	309	315	322	328	334
67	230	236	242	249	255	261	268	274	280	287	293	299	306	312	319	325	331	338	344
68	236	243	249	256	262	269	276	282	289	295	302	308	315	322	328	335	341	348	354
69	243	250	257	263	270	277	284	291	297	304	311	318	324	331	338	345	351	358	365
70	250	257	264	271	278	285	292	299	306	313	320	327	334	341	348	355	362	369	376
71	257	265	272	279	286	293	301	308	315	322	329	338	343	351	358	365	372	379	386
72	265	272	279	287	294	302	309	316	324	331	338	346	353	361	368	375	383	390	397
73	272	280	288	295	302	310	318	325	333	340	348	355	363	371	378	386	393	401	408
74	280	287	295	303	311	319	326	334	342	350	358	365	373	381	389	396	404	412	420
75	287	295	303	311	319	327	335	343	351	359	367	375	383	391	399	407	415	423	431
76	295	304	312	320	328	336	344	353	361	369	377	385	394	402	410	418	426	435	443

Your Body, Part by Part

Now that you know your body weight and BMI, it's time to tackle your waist circumference. Position a soft, flexible tape measure at the narrowest part of your trunk, just above your navel. Be sure to keep the tape level. You may be able to measure your waist yourself or you may need a little help. If you measure it alone, do so in front of a mirror, where you can make sure that the tape stays horizontal and straight. Record the number.

Take your BMI and your waist measurement, then check the table below. It will help you gauge your risk of weight-related health consequences. Women with a waist greater than 35 inches and men with a waist bigger than 40 inches face higher risk. That's a sign of more fat around the middle—pounds that are linked with a higher risk of type 2 diabetes, high blood pressure, heart disease, and metabolic syndrome (more on that below). Knowing your odds can help you decide how much effort you want to put into instilling your healthy new habits.

Some racial differences are emerging here, too. A growing number of scientists believe that people from Asian countries should aim for smaller waistlines—30 inches or less for women and 35 inches or less for men. That's because the risk of health problems seems to appear at those sizes, likely a reflection of more fat around the middle.

RATE YOUR WEIGHT, WAIST, AND RISK*

Body Mass Index (BMI)		Waist†	
		Men: < 40 inches	> 40 inches
		Women: < 35 inches	> 35 inches
Underweight	<18.5		
Healthy	18.5–24.9		
Overweight	25–29.9	Increased risk	High risk
		Men: < 40 inches	> 40 inches
		Women: < 35 inches	> 35 inches
Obese	30–34.9	High risk	Very high risk
Obese	35–39.9	Very high	Very high
Obese	40+	Extremely high	Extremely high

SOURCE: National Heart, Lung, and Blood Institute

*For type 2 diabetes, high blood pressure, and heart disease
†Asian men < 35 inches; Asian women < 30 inches

Whatever your results, it's also a smart idea to know the following: your blood pressure; blood triglyceride levels; fasting blood sugar; total blood cholesterol; and levels of high-density lipoprotein, the so-called good cholesterol.

An overweight or obese body mass index, plus three or more of the following risk factors, is a strong indicator that you are at high risk for metabolic syndrome, a condition that afflicts an estimated 47 million adults in the United States and places you at increased odds of developing diabetes and premature heart disease:

- Waistline: larger than 40 inches for men, 35 inches for women (larger than 35 inches for Asian men, 30 inches for Asian women)

- Blood pressure of 130/85 mm or higher

- Triglyceride level 150 mg/dL or more

- Fasting blood sugar measurement of more than 100 mg/dL

- Blood levels of the protective cholesterol, high-density lipoprotein (HDL), less than 40 mg/dL for men, less than 50 mg/dL for women

If you discover that you are prone to metabolic syndrome, don't panic. You can take steps to help reduce your risk. Be sure to consult with your doctor or other health professional for additional help.

And find inspiration from the experience of Arkansas governor Mike Huckabee. In 2002, he was diagnosed with type 2 diabetes. With the help of weight-loss doctors at the University of Arkansas for Medical Sciences in Little Rock, he began to change his eating and exercise habits. Governor Huckabee has lost more than 100 pounds over about a year—and reversed his diabetes in the process.

In 2004, I met Governor Huckabee at the *Time*/ABC News Obesity Summit in Williamsburg, Virginia, where we both were speakers. The governor eloquently described how he used to have trouble just walking around the block and now jogs several miles daily, rides a stationary bike while he reads the morning newspaper, and does strength training with weights. He's written a wonderful book about his weighty odyssey, *Quit Digging Your Grave with a Knife and Fork: A 12-Stop Program to End Bad Habits and Begin a Healthy Lifestyle*. Formerly obese and at risk for a premature death, Governor Huckabee now runs marathons, inspires others to achieve a healthier weight, and has become a Lean Plate Club member.

If Governor Huckabee, who also chairs the National Governors Association, can make these habit changes while in office—and see such significant health improvements—imagine what you can do, too, no matter how busy your schedule.

What's Likely to Work Best for You?

The following questions will help you assess whether reaching a healthier weight is something that you may do best on your own, with a friend, or with a larger group. Circle the number next to your answer. Use your score as a guide—not as an absolute—to help you consider various options.

1. I love getting help and encouragement from my family, friends, and colleagues when I'm trying to change habits.

   5   Right on!

   3   Yes, I like a little help.

   1   No way!

2. When I am trying to shed some pounds, I prefer to go it alone. No meddling, please!

   1   That describes me to a T.

   3   Yes, sometimes I do better when I'm mostly left to my own devices.

   5   Not a chance!

3. I hate counting calories, measuring food, and paying attention to portion sizes.

   1   My sentiments exactly.

   3   It's not my favorite activity, but I'll do it.

   5   Sure, bring on those measuring cups, spoons, and the kitchen scale. I'm ready.

4. Don't limit my food choices—just tell me that I can have a little bit of everything.

   5   Oh yeah, that's me.

   3   I'm okay with cutting out certain foods—sometimes.

   1   No way. Just tell me what to eat so I don't have to think too much about this.

Scoring: If you scored 12 or higher, you seem to like social support. Variety in food is also important, and you're willing to do the numbers. You may want to consider teaming with a family member, friend, or colleague—or even joining an organized weight-loss group (Weight Watchers, TOPS, Food Addicts) for some additional help with your efforts. If you scored less than 12, you seem to prefer tackling this problem on your own. You may want to consider trying one of the self-help books or Internet-based programs, including the online Lean Plate Club weekly Web chat, for more private support of your efforts.

STEP 4: ARE YOU READY TO BE MORE ACTIVE?

Nothing takes the place of a thorough physical exam by your physician or health-care provider. So if you have not had a physical in more than a year, it is a good idea to schedule one, especially if you have any chronic medical problems or if your weight has changed significantly in the past year.

In the meantime, the British Columbia Ministry of Health in Canada has developed a widely used questionnaire, called the PAR-Q test, designed to screen people ages 15 to 69 years for their readiness to be physically active.

PAR-Q & YOU

The Canadian Society for Exercise Physiology, Health Canada, and their agents assume no liability for persons who undertake physical activity, and if in doubt after completing this questionnaire, consult your doctor prior to physical activity.

Informed use of the PAR-Q: The Canadian Society for Exercise Physiology, Health Canada, and their agents assume no liability for persons who undertake physical activity, and if in doubt after completing this questionnaire, consult your doctor prior to physical activity. Note: This physical activity clearance is valid for a maximum of 12 months from the date it is completed and becomes invalid if your condition changes so that you would answer *yes* to any of the seven questions.

Regular physical activity is fun and healthy, and increasingly more people are starting to become more active every day. Being more active is very safe for most people. However, some people should check with their doctor before they start becoming much more physically active.

If you are planning to become much more physically active than you are now, start by answering the seven questions below. If you are between the ages of 15 and 69, the PAR-Q will tell you if you should check with your doctor before you start. If you are over 69 years of age, and you are not used to being very active, check with your doctor.

Common sense is your best guide when you answer these questions. Please read the questions carefully and answer each one honestly: Check *yes* or *no*.

YES	NO		
☐	☐	1.	Has your doctor ever said that you have a heart condition *and* that you should only do physical activity recommended by a doctor?
☐	☐	2.	Do you feel pain in your chest when you do physical activity?
☐	☐	3.	In the past month, have you had chest pain when you were not doing physical activity?
☐	☐	4.	Do you lose your balance because of dizziness or do you ever lose consciousness?
☐	☐	5.	Do you have a bone or joint problem (for example, back, knee, or hip) that could be made worse by a change in your physical activity?

(continued)

☐   ☐   6. Is your doctor currently prescribing drugs (for example, water pills) for your blood pressure or heart condition?

☐   ☐   7. Do you know of *any other reason* why you should not do physical activity?

If you answered yes to one or more questions:

Talk with your doctor by phone or in person *before* you start becoming much more physically active or *before* you have a fitness appraisal. Tell your doctor about the PAR-Q and which questions you answered *yes*.

- You may be able to do any activity you want—as long as you start slowly and build up gradually. Or, you may need to restrict your activities to those which are safe for you. Talk with your doctor about the kinds of activities you wish to participate in and follow his/her advice.

- Find out which community programs are safe and helpful for you.

If you answered *no* to all questions:

If you answered *no* honestly to *all* PAR-Q questions, you can be reasonably sure that you can:

- Start becoming much more physically active—begin slowly and build up gradually. This is the safest and easiest way to go.

- Take part in a fitness appraisal—this is an excellent way to determine your basic fitness so that you can plan the best way for you to live actively. It is also highly recommended that you have your blood pressure evaluated. If your reading is over

144/94, talk with your doctor before you start becoming much more physically active.

↓
Delay becoming much more active:

• If you are not feeling well because of temporary illness such as a cold or a fever—wait until you feel better; or

• If you may be pregnant—talk to your doctor before you start becoming more active.

Source: Physical Activity Readiness Questionnaire (PAR-Q). Copyright © 2002. Reprinted with permission of the Canadian Society for Exercise Physiology, Inc. http://www.csep.ca/forms.asp.

Please note: If your health changes so that you then answer *yes* to any of the above questions, tell your fitness or health professional. Ask whether you should change your physical activity plan.

Three

SETTING YOUR GOALS AND HOW TO GET THERE

Each week on the Lean Plate Club Web chat, I get questions like these:

Hi, Sally: I hope you can help. I'm 35, sit at a desk most of the day, but do manage to get out for about a half-hour walk on most days. I usually go with a friend. We've just started doing this. I want to lose about ten pounds. How much should I eat daily?

Sally, I don't understand it. I've been jogging a mile every night after work and have joined a gym, where I go about twice a week. I'm not counting calories, but I know I'm eating better. I've even given up drinking a soft drink every afternoon. So how come I've only lost about a pound? I've been doing this for two weeks. It's so discouraging. I never had any trouble losing weight in college.

Hey, Sally: My fiftieth birthday is coming up later this year. I've vowed that I'm going to get rid of some of these extra pounds that I've put on through the years. I'm six feet tall, weigh 250 pounds, and spend a lot of time either at my desk or traveling for my job. I find it especially hard to eat well on the road. What's a reasonable calorie goal for me to lose weight?

HOW MANY CALORIES DAILY?

It's one of the first questions that those new to the Lean Plate Club ask. The answer depends on your age, gender, and activity level. If you're a desk jockey and rarely find time to take a walk, then you likely lead a mostly sedentary life, which means you need fewer calories daily than an active construction worker, nurse, waitress, bartender, flight attendant, or other professional who spends a lot of time on his or her feet during the workday. Here's what you need to know.

What's Moderate Physical Activity?

Bicycling (< 10 mph)

Dancing

Golf (walk/carry clubs)

Hiking

Light gardening/yard work

Stretching

Walking (3.5 mph or 17-minute miles)

Weight lifting

SOURCE: U.S. Centers for Disease Control and Prevention

Figure your activity level. Most of us overestimate this, so be realistic and honest. Consider all your daily activities, from what you do on the job, on your commute, and at home.

- *Sedentary:* You get less than 30 minutes daily of moderate physical activity. That means you're doing only the light physical activity associated with modern life, such as walking to your car in the parking lot, taking out the garbage, loading the dishwasher, walking up and down the stairs in your house. (Yes, this is the majority of us.)

- *Moderately active:* You manage to do at least 30 to 60 minutes daily of moderate activity—that's equal to walking one and one-half to three miles per day at a pace of three to four miles per hour, or hoofing about a mile in no more than 15 minutes. That exercise is in addition to the light activities of daily life, such as doing the laundry, walking to the cafeteria, sweeping your front steps, or bringing groceries from the car. So maybe you walk at lunch, bike to work, take a morning jog, or participate in an aerobics class on most days.

- *Active:* You make an effort to get 60 minutes or more of moderate physical activity in addition to your regular schedule on most days. This means walking briskly (about four miles per hour or 15-minute miles). It could be fast-paced morning and evening constitutionals with your dog, a noon game of pickup basketball every weekday, a daily five-mile run, or a spinning class on most days at your gym with long hikes on the weekend. Again, this activity is in addition to what you do in the normal course of daily life.

Determine how many calories you need to maintain your current weight. The Institute of Medicine, an arm of the National Academy of Sciences in Washington, D.C., offers the guidelines on page 59 for daily energy intake. The numbers provided give you calorie levels based on your activity and your age. They're a ballpark estimate required to maintain your current weight.

BOOST ACTIVITY, EAT A LITTLE MORE

Sedentary (S)
(less than 30 minutes per day of moderate physical activity in addition to daily activities)

Moderately Active (MA)
(between 30 and 60 minutes per day of moderate physical activity in addition to daily activities)

Active (A)
(60 minutes per day of moderate physical activity in addition to daily activities)

	Men				Women		
Age	S	MA	A	Age	S	MA	A
18	2,400	2,800	3,200	18	2,000	2,000	2,400
19–20	2,600	2,800	3,000	19–20	2,000	2,200	2,400
21–25	2,400	2,800	3,000	21–25	2,000	2,200	2,400
26–30	2,400	2,600	3,000	26–30	1,800	2,000	2,400
31–35	2,400	2,600	3,000	31–35	1,800	2,000	2,200
36–40	2,400	2,600	2,800	36–40	1,800	2,000	2,200
41–45	2,200	2,600	2,800	41–45	1,800	2,000	2,200
46–50	2,200	2,400	2,800	46–50	1,800	2,000	2,200
51–55	2,200	2,400	2,800	51–55	1,600	1,800	2,200
56–60	2,200	2,400	2,600	56–60	1,600	1,800	2,200
61–65	2,000	2,400	2,600	61–65	1,600	1,800	2,000
71–75	2,000	2,200	2,600	71–75	1,600	1,800	2,000
76 and older	2,000	2,200	2,400	76 and older	1,600	1,800	2,000

SOURCES: Institute of Medicine Dietary Reference Intakes Macronutrients Report, 2002; USDA Center for Nutrition Policy and Promotion, April 2005

Do the math. Weight loss, of course, requires some calorie adjustment. To lose one pound per week means achieving a deficit of about 500 calories a day. You can do that a number of ways, but one of the easiest, safest, and most pleasant ways is with a combination of less food and more activity. Simply cut back on 250 calories of food per day—the equivalent of forgoing one 20-ounce bottle of a soft drink—and get 250 more calories of activity daily—equal to a brisk 40-minute walk. Do that daily, and in a week, it adds up to a 3,500-calorie deficit or a one-pound weight loss.

	DAILY CALORIE DEFICITS	
	Less food	**More activity**
To lose:		
(pound/week)		
½	125	125
1	250	250
1½	375	375
2	500	500

Another option is simply to look at the bottom line. Leading university-based weight-loss clinics start women on 1,200 to 1,500 calories a day to lose weight and put men on 1,500 to 1,800 calories a day.

To lose ½ pound per week:

Your daily calories _____

                               –250 calories (reduce food/day)

                Total: _____

To lose 1 pound:

Your daily calories _____

                               –250 calories (reduce food/day)

                               –250 calories (increase activity/day)

                Total: _____

To cut calories or stay within daily calorie limits, you'll need to measure, track, record, and count what you eat. Studies show that most people are notoriously bad at doing that. It also turns out that the heavier you are, the worse you are at correctly gauging what you eat. Studies suggest that lean people underestimate their daily calories by about 20 percent. Overweight people underestimate their calories by 40 percent. That can add up to a whole lot of unexpected calories.

You can take the guesswork out of calorie counting by measuring what you eat. Get out your measuring cups and spoons. Place them in a very accessible spot in your kitchen. And consider having a couple of sets of measuring cups and spoons so that when one is dirty, you've got another one to grab. Ideally, get a set that has measurements down to one-eighth of a cup and one-eighth of a teaspoon. **Here's the secret: Using them will help you keep portions under control. While you have them handy, use them to gauge the sizes of your most commonly used glasses, cups, dishes, and ramekins.** Fill a one-cup container with water and pour into various glasses and bowls. You may be surprised to learn that they hold either a lot more or a lot less than you think.

Did that slice of salmon you ate weigh three ounces or six? How about that pork chop?

The most accurate way to gauge portion size is by measuring food. While cups and spoons can be helpful, only a scale can tell you exactly how much that chicken breast weighs. Roundups of the latest in kitchen scales, which start at about $10, are available at www.epinions.com.

A kitchen scale is another essential tool for your healthy new habits. Scales come in all shapes, sizes, and styles. They begin at about $20 and are well worth the investment. Get one that is easy to read and can be zeroed for better accuracy. "I still weigh and measure almost everything," says a Lean Plate Club member who has shed 150 pounds since January 2001 with a combination of Weight Watchers and the Lean Plate Club. "Even when I make pasta, I weigh it first before I put it in the water to make sure that I am having just one portion."

While you're at it, pick up some disposable containers at the grocery store in half-cup and one-cup sizes. They're great for leftovers, of course, but **here's the secret: Use them for quick measurements or to pack healthy snacks or lunch on the go in premeasured sizes.** Some Lean Plate Club members also save the portioned plates from frozen dinners. They wash them and use them as a quick way to gauge portion sizes for another meal.

When you're in the kitchen, take a close look around:

- Do you keep tempting food on the counter that makes it easy to reach and eat? Move it out of sight or get rid of it altogether.

• What foods are in your pantry that might undermine your efforts? Consider donating them to a food shelter, taking them to your church, synagogue, or mosque for use, or sharing them with your coworkers. Do a similar check of your freezer and refrigerator.

THE WELL-STOCKED LEAN PLATE CLUB KITCHEN

Habits don't change overnight, and neither do kitchens. So here's a list of kitchen staples to begin stocking as you add healthier habits to achieve a healthier weight. No need to purchase all of these items at once—or ever. This list is merely a starting point. Be guided by your taste preferences and those of your family, as well as what fits your budget.

Pantry/Cupboards

Broths and Soups *(low sodium where possible, since you can always add more flavoring including salt; preferably without cream)*
Beef bouillon and broth
Black bean
Chicken
Chicken noodle
Lentil
Manhattan clam chowder
Minestrone
Miso (high in sodium for those counting sodium milligrams)
Mushroom
No-Chicken Chicken Broth (made from vegetables but tastes like chicken)
Tomato
Vegetable

Cereals
Oatmeal
Whole-grain, unsweetened ready-to-eat cereal

Chocolate
Semisweet or unsweetened chocolate
Unsweetened cocoa

Crackers
Ak-Mak
flatbreads
Ryvita
Triscuits
Wasa
Whole wheat matzo

Flour
Specialty flours such as peanut, garbanzo, rice flour, and others
Unbleached white
Whole wheat

Nuts/Seeds (slivered, when possible)
Almonds
Cashews
Peanuts
Pecans
Sesame
Walnuts

Oil
Canola oil
Canola oil spray

Olive oil spray
Peanut oil
Safflower oil
Sesame oil (light or dark)
Sunflower oil
Virgin olive oil
Walnut oil

Pasta/Noodles/Rice/Whole Grains

Basmati rice
Brown rice (Uncle Ben's and Success make quicker-cooking
    brown rice, but you can also buy frozen cooked brown rice.)
Bulgur wheat
Couscous, whole wheat
Penne, multigrain (Barilla Plus Penne made *Health* magazine's
    2005 list of Best Foods: It contains egg whites, lentils,
    chickpeas, and flaxseeds to boost fiber and protein content.)
Popcorn
Quinoa
Spaghetti (white and/or whole wheat)
White rice
Wild rice (Find cooked wild rice in vacuum packets at Trader
    Joe's, a specialty grocery in many states.)

Sauces

Green sauce for Mexican food
Low-fat Alfredo
Marinara
Salsa
Simmer sauces
Tomato

Vegetables (preferably low sodium or no added sodium, so you can flavor according to your taste)
Beans (black, kidney, garbanzo, white, red, pink, etc.)
Carrots
Lentils
Pumpkin
Sweet potatoes
Tomatoes
Tomato juice
Tomato paste
V8 or other vegetable juice
Water chestnuts

Condiments and Vinegar
Balsamic vinegar (red or white)
Ketchup
Mustard
Orange muscat champagne vinegar (or other specialty vinegars)
Raspberry vinegar
Red wine vinegar
Rice vinegar (lite)
Soy sauce (reduced sodium)
Tabasco
White vinegar
Worcestershire sauce

Jellies/Jams/"Butters"
Almond butter
Apple butter
Fruit spreads without added sugar
Peanut butter
Pumpkin butter

Fish
Anchovies
Kippers
Salmon
Sardines
Tuna

Fruit
Apple, pear, or other "sauces," unsweetened (Santa Cruz Organic
    Apple Blackberry Sauce snagged a 2005 Excellence in Food
    Award from *Health* magazine.)
Blueberry, cranberry, pomegranate, or other unsweetened juices
    (Walnut Acres Organic Blueberry Juice also made *Health*
    magazine's 2005 list of Best Foods.)
Cans, jars, or cups of fruit in its own juice
Dried fruit

Dessert
Puddings

Refrigerator

Dairy
Fat-free or low-fat cheese (especially Laughing Cow, partially
    skim mozzarella, Parmesan, nonfat feta and other low-fat
    goat cheese, string cheese, and cottage cheese; fat-free cream
    cheese and sour cream. (Cabot Creamery 75% Light
    Vermont Cheddar made *Health* magazine's 2005 list of Best
    Foods)
Nonfat or low-fat milk (lactose reduced for those with lactose
    intolerance)
Nonfat or low-fat plain yogurt (especially Total Greek yogurt by
    Fage)

Soy milk (Silk Enhanced Soymilk, plain, grabbed a 2005 Best
    Foods Award from *Health* magazine. It contains folic acid;
    healthy omega-3 fatty acids; vitamins A, C, and E; and calcium.)

Eggs
Egg substitutes or egg whites for those watching cholesterol
    levels
Whole eggs

Fruit
As many varieties and colors as you like

Seeds
Flaxseeds (to grind on salads or put in baked goods)

Fish
Any fresh fish
Pickled herring
Smoked salmon

Margarines/Spreads/Garnishes
Benecol or Take Control (which have cholesterol-lowering
    stanols and sterols)
Capers
Dill pickles
Fat-free or reduced-fat sour cream
Horseradish
Hot/sweet pickled peppers
Mayonnaise (light or reduced fat if possible)
Olives
Pickled okra
Smart Balance
Tub or stick margarines (without trans fat), such as Promises

Meat/Meat Substitutes/Poultry

Chicken or turkey sausage
Leanest cuts of meat
Poultry (remove skin)
Seitan
Tempeh
Tofu
Turkey bacon

Freezer

Frozen dinners (Lean Cuisine Spa Cuisine and Amy's Indian
   Mattar Paneer snagged spots on the Best Foods list of *Health*
   magazine.)
Frozen waffles, whole grain and low fat
Lean cuts of beef, pork, lamb
Meatless burgers, "hot dogs," or meat substitutes, especially Boca
   Burgers (The Boca Cheeseburger made the 2005 Best Foods
   list of *Health* magazine.)
Skinless chicken or turkey breast and/or thighs
Tortellini
Unsweetened fruit
Vegetables without sauces that contain fat or sodium, including
   spinach, broccoli, peas, carrots, French string beans

Desserts

Nonfat or low-fat ice cream
Skinny Cow by Silhouette
Sorbet

FOOD RECORDS

Having a well-stocked kitchen so that you can cook healthful, good-tasting food is one step. Measuring what you eat is another while you're gradually restocking your pantry, fridge, and freezer.

Also important to instilling your healthy new habits is to record what you eat. That's essential to get an accurate idea of your daily intake—and the only way to be sure that you aren't experiencing calorie creep, the insidious rise of daily calories.

Will you have to record what you eat forever? Probably not. But it's a very valuable habit for these early weeks. And recording food also comes in handy from time to time as a check to be sure that you're not drifting upward calorically.

Some Lean Plate Club members use their daily pocket calendars to record their food. Others buy a journal just for this purpose. You can carry a little notebook with you in a shirt pocket, your purse, or your briefcase. You can photocopy the food record on page 73 and use that. Or you can use one of the growing number of electronic tools that will do the numbers for you on your desktop, laptop, or PDA. These are just a few of the resources available to take the guesswork out of calorie counting for the next few weeks. Some people find that's all the time it takes for them to get their portion sizes under control and to find the right caloric bal-

- Load leftovers into single-serving-size containers, ready to grab the next day for lunch.
- Measure tempting snack foods—chips, peanuts, pretzels—into single-size plastic bags to help put the brakes on nonstop eating.
- Reserve a "grab-and-go" place in your refrigerator, cupboard, or pantry. Stock it with prepared, premeasured food.

Smart snack choices:
- Baby carrots with low-fat ranch dressing
- Cut-up fruit
- "Antipasto" with slices of red pepper, olives, and celery
- Half-cup containers of tabouleh
- Hummus or baba ghanoush

---

ance. For others, measuring food and tracking calories needs to be a longer habit. You're the best judge of what works well for you.

The point is to find a way to track what you eat in a fashion that suits you.

Here's a secret: If you can plan at least a meal in advance— better yet, a day ahead—it will help keep you a step ahead in healthy eating. When you already have food for your next meal planned or even prepared, you can better keep hunger at bay with regular meals. Some Lean Plate Club members find it helpful to cook a few meals ahead on weekends or double a recipe during the week to be sure there are leftovers for another meal. Some plan the next day's meals the night before so they don't find themselves scrounging for food when they come home from work tired and hungry.

You can also stock your desk—or car—with healthy fare. That reduces the risk that you'll grab the latest high-calorie offering at the office—or head to the vending machines—when you're stressed or hungry and can't leave for a more balanced meal. It should also keep you from noshing unhealthy stuff on the way home.

Throughout the Lean Plate Club Program, you'll find tips from experts as well as Lean Plate Club members who have discovered simple secrets that will help you succeed.

Desk Rations

Stock your desk with some healthy food and drink to reduce the temptation to hit the vending machines or grab something to eat that may cause regret later. Here are some possibilities:

- Premeasured ounce of nuts
- Soup (canned, dehydrated, or bouillon cubes)
- Sugarless gum
- Tea bags (with packet of lemon and packet of honey)
- Packet of hot chocolate
- Tuna pouch (Starkist)
- Fruit cups (mixed fruit, applesauce)
- V8
- Fruit rollup
- Single bag of microwave popcorn
- Dried fruit
- Energy, protein, or cereal bar

Amount	Calories	Fruit/Vegetable	Time Eaten
Breakfast			
Lunch			
Dinner			
Snacks			
Total			

Calorie-Counting Resources

Available free of charge unless otherwise indicated. Note: Prices are subject to change.

- **Balancelog,** www.healthetech.com. Free 14-day trial; $49 for software for PC and Palm; $29 for PDA alone.
- **Dallas Dietetics Association,** www.dallasdietitian.com/calcalc.htm. Offers an online calculator for figuring daily calories needed.
- **Diet Power,** www.dietpower.com. Free 15-day trial; $49.99 for download; $59.99 for CD-ROM.
- **The Doctor's Pocket Calorie, Fat & Carbohydrate Counter,** www.calorieking.com. $6.99 plus free downloads; Desktop Diet Diary, $29.95.
- **Fitday,** www.fitday.com. Free Web-based diet and fitness journal. Records intake and activity. Provides charts of calorie breakdowns. $29.95 for downloadable PC version; $39.95 for downloadable PC version plus CD-ROM.
- **My Food Diary,** www.myfooddiary.com. A food diary, exercise log, charts, and reports for $9/month.
- **MyPyramid Tracker,** www.mypyramidtracker.gov. The U.S. Department of Agriculture's tool for tracking up to a year's worth of food and physical activity records. Password protected.
- **Nutrition Data,** www.nutritiondata.com. Graphs your intake on a colorful pyramid that has the healthiest foods on the bottom, higher-calorie fare on the top. Provides extensive nutritional information about each food, as well as a long list of healthier choices. A fullness factor will guide you to filling but less caloric and more nutritious options.
- **Nutridiary,** www.nutridiary.com. Records food and exercise. Provides colorful analysis and charts of what you've eaten and offers a place to keep an online private journal about your quest for a healthier weight.

- **Nutrition Analysis Tools and System (NATS)**, http://nat.crgq.com. Free if used online; download to Palm-based PDA for $7.95.
- **Spark People,** www.sparkpeople.com. $1.99/week; billed quarterly; cancel at any time with unused weeks refundable.
- **South Beach Diet,** www.southbeachdiet.com. $5/week; billed quarterly; cancel at any time with unused weeks refundable except for a minimum $20 charge.
- **Weight Watchers,** www.weightwatchers.com. $16.95/month plus $29.95 sign-up fee; three-month savings plan $5/week plus $29.95 sign-up fee.

WHERE DO YOU GO FROM HERE?

You have a couple of options:

Option 1. Begin today. Jump ahead to Week 1 of the Lean Plate Club Program and plunge right in. The first week involves increasing your intake of fruit and vegetables and learning to stay within the daily calorie range for your goals. It will also prepare you to become more active. Come back at another time to read the next two chapters on nutrition and physical activity. They are designed to be read in easily digestible "bites"—without any added calories!—and will help ground you in the basics of nutrition and physical activity so that you'll never be beholden to the next food or exercise fad to come along.

Option 2. Set a date to begin within the next week. Write it on your calendar. Let your family, significant other, roommate, friends, or colleagues know about your efforts as you feel appropriate. In the meantime, the next two chapters will give you basics on nutrition and physical activity. You can read them now or in the days ahead. You'll learn how to take stock of your favorite healthy foods and physical activity.

Whichever way you choose, throughout these pages you'll find plenty of inspiration from Lean Plate Club members. Like you, some are at the beginning of their quest for healthier habits. Others have achieved their goals and now are focused on maintaining their healthy weight. And still others fall somewhere in between. It's now completely up to you how you move forward to add these secrets to your own life.

Four

NUTRITION BITE BY BITE

Before you started to read, you had to learn the alphabet. Before you could count, you needed to know a little bit about numbers. Even as a child, before you played dodgeball or kickball on the playground, you learned the rules.

The same is true today. You consult a manual to program your VCR, DVD player, or Tivo. You likely seek technical assistance for your computer, Internet connection, MP3 player, or cell phone. And you wouldn't think of dealing a hand of Texas hold 'em poker without first learning the rules of play.

So why would you think that just because you've eaten food all your life, you should have some innate, expert knowledge of nutrition? Yet without that knowledge, you're at the mercy of every food fad and nutritional myth that comes along.

Here's what you need to know.

PROTEIN

In high school biology, you learned that protein is one of those essential nutrients that we all need to live. That's because protein, which comes from the Greek word *proteios*, meaning "primary," serves as the major structural component for every cell in the body. That's right—every cell in the body.

And if that weren't enough, protein also is a key part of numerous chemicals that make the body function like a well-oiled machine. Protein forms hemoglobin that allows red blood cells to carry oxygen throughout the body. Without protein, there wouldn't be muscle or collagen, both of which provide the scaffolding for skin and bone. Protein is required to make estrogen, testosterone, and numerous other hormones, including insulin that ferries sugar into cells for energy. And protein serves as the cellular equivalent to homeland security, setting up checkpoints in each cell's outer membrane to dictate what gets in and out.

The latest evidence suggests another benefit of protein. Turns out that it is better than either carbohydrates or fats at promoting satiety—that is, helping you to feel full. Learn more about how best to add protein in Week 4.

Before you fret about getting enough protein, know this: Protein comes in everything from meat, poultry, seafood, eggs, and dairy products to beans and nuts. Even foods that you might not think of as protein sources have a little of it, including bread, dates, and oatmeal.

Odds are that you're already getting enough for nutritional purposes. In fact, large national nutrition surveys conducted by the U.S. Department of Agriculture show that protein deficiency is rarely a problem in the United States or other developed countries where food is plentiful and populations are generally overnourished. Vegans, who eat no animal products, are the rare exception. They need to be vigilant to get sufficient protein from varied plant sources.

So how much protein do you need every day? If you want to do the math down to the gram of protein, you can, but there's no need to do so. A chicken breast will likely give you the five and a half ounces or so of protein that you need daily. So will a salmon steak, a large pork chop, a couple of small lamb chops, or about one and a half cups of beans or tofu. So will a cup of bean chili and a peanut butter sandwich.

Protein

What the experts say: Men need about 56 grams daily; women need about 46 grams a day. That's about 5 to 6 ounces of protein, about the amount found in a chicken breast or a salmon steak.

If you want to do the math:

Your body weight (pounds) _____
Multiply by 0.37 = grams protein/day.

Example: A 175-pound person × 0.37 = 65 grams, or the amount found in three glasses of skim milk, a chicken breast, and a bean burrito.

SOURCE: National Academy of Sciences Dietary References Intake Macronutrient Report

---

If you want more specifics, the National Academy of Sciences recommends 56 grams of protein daily for men and 46 grams for women, based on a 154-pound man and a 127-pound woman. (If your weight is significantly different, the numbers may change a little.)

To put the numbers in perspective, four ounces of shrimp and a pork chop (without the bone) each have about half a day's worth of protein, as do three glasses of skim milk. Two bean burritos with cheese and a cup of beans have 75 percent of the protein women need, more than half that needed by men. Two scrambled eggs provide about a quarter of the daily recommended protein intake while a one-pound porterhouse steak has a whopping 106 grams of protein—or more than double the daily recommendation for most people—plus 105 grams of fat, 42 of them unhealthy saturated fat. You get the picture. For more information on protein, see Week 4 of the Lean Plate Club Program.

HOW MUCH PROTEIN?		
Age (years)	Men (ounces)*	Women (ounces)*
19–30	6½	5½
31–50	6	5
51+	5½	5

SOURCE: USDA

*1 ounce of protein = 1 ounce of lean meat, poultry, or fish; 1 egg; 1 tablespoon of peanut butter; ¼ ounce of cooked dried beans; ½ ounce of nuts or seeds.

CARBOHYDRATES

They've been demonized in recent years, castigated by a number of popular diets from Atkins to Sugar Busters to South Beach. There's no question that many people have overindulged in carbohydrates, especially highly processed carbs, made with white flour, little fiber, and plenty of added sugar. They've guzzled megaportions of sweetened soft drinks with enough calories for an entire day. They've gorged on boxes of sugary fat-free cookies, mistakenly believing that no fat is equivalent to low-calorie. They've started the day with white bread toast, bagels, and sugar-coated cereals that are as sweet as dessert only to find themselves famished again by midmorning.

Those who either eat the most highly processed carbs or drastically cut back on carbs miss a great opportunity. Carbohydrates are an essential nutrient that is every bit as important as protein, healthy fat, and various key vitamins and minerals.

Shortchange carbohydrates and the brain may not get enough glucose—the simple sugar that is the preferred fuel for cells in the brain and the central nervous system. And by the way, glucose is also the only fuel that red blood cells can use.

So how does the body compensate when there aren't enough carbs to produce sufficient glucose? Simple. It breaks down fat, muscle, and other tissue to keep the brain fueled. Known as ketosis, in this process the body cannibalizes its own tissues to preserve the brain.

Carbohydrates

Make healthy carbs about half your daily calories:*

2 cups fruit

2½ cups vegetables

3–6 servings whole grains

1 serving =

1 slice whole-grain bread;

1 cup ready-to-eat whole grain cereal;

½ cup cooked whole grains, whole-grain pasta, whole-grain cereal

3 cups of fat-free or low-fat milk or other dairy food

What you need: 130 grams of carbohydrates daily for brain function. That's equal to about 2 large pieces of fruit plus 3 slices of whole wheat bread.

SOURCES: 2005 Dietary Guidelines Committee Report; National Academy of Sciences Dietary Reference Intakes Energy, Carbohydrate, Fiber, Fat, Fatty Acids, Cholesterol, Protein, and Amino Acids

*Based on 2,000 calories daily

After an exhaustive review of the latest scientific literature, the National Academy of Sciences set 130 grams per day as the recommended dietary allowance (RDA) for carbohydrates. The RDA is the average daily intake needed to meet the nutrient requirements of nearly all healthy adults and children.

Most people think of carbohydrates simply as starch, but that doesn't begin to do them justice. Carbs offer a cornucopia of possibilities. In fact, fruit and vegetables are among the healthiest carbohydrates you can eat—unless, of course, you deep-fat fry them, coat them with lots of added sugar, or drown them in butter or oil. The complex carbohydrates in fruits and vegetables are broken down slowly by the body and so don't spike blood sugar or insulin levels the way that simpler, more processed sugars do. In addition, fruits and vegetables come loaded with essential vitamins and minerals, fiber, and a variety of health-promoting phytonutrients, from lycopene and lutein to quercetin and a whole lot more.

Healthy carbs also include whole grains, whether they come baked in a crusty loaf of whole wheat or ladled out in a steamy bowl of oatmeal. Shredded wheat, brown rice, Triscuits, and even popcorn are just a few of the whole-grain healthy carbs that make smart choices.

And then there's dairy. Besides being a good source of protein and calcium, milk and other dairy products provide healthy carbs. Mostly this comes from lactose, a sugar that doesn't taste sweet and doesn't spike blood sugar levels or boost insulin production as much as more processed sugars, including glucose or sucrose. Even though it's a healthy carbohydrate, lactose isn't easily digested by those who lack the enzyme needed to break it down, a condition called lactose intolerance. If you're one of the 30 to 50 million Americans with this condition, nonprescription lactase enzyme tablets and liquids are available to help digest lactose. Lactose-reduced milk and other dairy products are also widely available at supermarkets.

These days, no discussion of healthy carbohydrates would be complete without mention of the glycemic index. The 2005 Dietary Guidelines Advisory Committee Report includes a section on the glycemic index. The bestselling *South Beach Diet* also takes into account the glycemic index of food, as do a number of other well-known diet tomes, including *Sugar Busters, Eat Yourself Slim, The Perricone Prescription*, and *Glycemic Index Diet*.

So what exactly is the glycemic index?

Simply this: The glycemic index (GI) calculates how fast blood sugar rises and stays elevated for two hours after food or drink is consumed. GI ratings are then compared against blood sugar scores for eating either pure glucose or white bread. Food and drink that score below the GI for glucose or white bread are classified as low glycemic; scores above glucose or white bread are high glycemic.

Should you even care about the glycemic index? Some respected scientists believe that eating according to the glycemic index may be a smart compromise between low-fat and low-carb regimens, since doing so doesn't require severe restriction of either fat or carbohydrates. Not everyone agrees, although with 17 million people suffering from diabetes in the United States alone, the glycemic index is getting a closer look from scientists, physicians, and the public.

To date, studies show mixed results on whether a low-glycemic regimen helps reduce weight. It has not been proved that eating a low-glycemic diet reduces the risk of diabetes, or that there are other health benefits of a low-glycemic approach. Among the possible benefits of a lower glycemic diet: reduction of triglycerides, an unhealthy type of blood fat; reduced risk of cancer; higher levels of high-density lipoprotein (HDL), a protective type of cholesterol; and lower levels of C-reactive protein, a marker of inflammation that is associated with increased heart disease risk, rheumatoid arthritis, rheumatic fever, and other conditions. It's still under investigation.

The 2005 Dietary Guidelines Advisory Committee concluded that "current evidence [indicates] that the glycemic index and/or glycemic load are of little utility for providing dietary guidance for Americans." The committee noted that following a low-glycemic-index regimen may help reduce blood sugar levels after eating but concluded that "there is not sufficient evidence of long term benefit to recommend general use of diets that have a low-glycemic index."

The secret is this: You can drive yourself crazy by religiously ferreting out the glycemic index of every food you eat.
For now, most nutrition experts—including even some propo-
nents studying the glycemic index—say that there's no need to
play the numbers game until the details are sorted out.

If you want to hedge your bets, **here's the secret: Skip highly
processed foods with minimal amounts of fiber and lots of
added sugar.** Instead, eat plenty of fruits and vegetables, whole
grains, low-fat milk and dairy products, as well as low-fat protein
and healthy fat, from avocados, nuts, and olive oil. Doing that will
keep you on the low end of the glycemic index without bothering
to count GI scores.

Eat Daily

Use this form to plan your daily fare.

_____ cups fruit (fresh, frozen, canned, or dried)

_____ cups vegetables (fresh, frozen, canned, or dried)

_____ servings of grains (half as whole grains)*

Three 8-ounce glasses of milk (or dairy equivalent)

_____ ounces lean meat, fish, or poultry without skin; tofu or
meat substitute; or _____ cups of cooked beans; or _____
tablespoons peanut butter. (1½ ounces of nuts or 1 egg also equals
the protein in 1 ounce of meat.)

_____ teaspoons healthy oil (olive, canola, safflower, sunflower,
peanut), mayonnaise, healthy margarine (without trans fats)

SOURCE: 2005 U.S. Dietary Guidelines

*1 serving = 1 slice bread, ½ cup rice, or 1 cup ready-to-eat cereal.

FAT

It used to be a dirty word, with a terrible reputation. Less than a decade ago, fat-free foods jammed grocery shelves and consumers ate them with abandon, foolishly thinking that no fat means no calories.

The truth is that all fat is not created equal. So think of fat as the slightly edgy essential nutrient, the one that looks seductive, tastes great, and yet—depending on how smart you choose—can leave you feeling virtuous or guilty. All fat contains nine calories per gram, more than twice the calories of either protein or carbohydrates. Indulge too much in any type of fat and you risk gaining weight. Eat too little fat and you may not be able to absorb enough vitamins A, D, E, and K, which are important for everything from fighting infection to preserving bones.

Eat Weekly

2 servings seafood

3 cups cooked, dried beans (baked beans, bean soup, bean salads, etc.)

3 cups dark green vegetables (spinach, collard and mustard greens, kale, etc.)

2 cups orange vegetables (carrots, sweet potatoes, pumpkin, peppers, etc.)

3 cups starchy vegetables (corn, potatoes, etc.)

6½ cups other vegetables (lettuce, eggplant, tomatoes, broccoli, cabbage, Brussels sprouts, onions, etc.)

SOURCES: 2005 U.S. Dietary Guidelines; National Cancer Institute's 5 to 9 a Day program; American Heart Association

---

There's also been a misunderstanding of the terms "low fat" and "moderate fat," which are sometimes used interchangeably. Suffice it to say that the current nutritional consensus is to keep fats at about a fifth (20 percent) to up to about a third (35 percent) of your daily calories. (If you eat 2,000 calories a day, that works out to 400–700 calories or 44–78 grams of fat. Foodwise, that equals the fat found in a small cheeseburger with chips, an egg, and a couple of pats of margarine.)

Despite some confusion about fat, what hasn't changed is the importance of limiting unhealthy fat, which can help clog arteries and increases the risk of breast, colon, and prostate cancer, as well as other tumors. A simple rule of thumb: At room temperature, unhealthy fat is solid, while healthy fats are liquid or oils. It all has to do with chemistry. Here's what leading medical, nutrition, and government health groups recommend.

- **Saturated fat.** Mostly found in animal products such as butter, fatty cuts of meat, poultry skin, bacon, lard, tallow, shortening, marbled cuts of meat, many stick margarines, cheese, and full-fat dairy products. Coconut and palm kernel oil are two plant-based sources of saturated fat. No matter where it originates, saturated fat helps raise blood levels of low-density lipoprotein (LDL), one of the most damaging types of blood cholesterol. **Advice:** Eat 10 percent or less total calories from saturated fat. If you already have symptoms of heart disease, then limit saturated fat to 7 percent or less of daily calories. On 2,000 calories daily, that works out to 200 calories or 22 grams of fat. In fast-food fare, that's equal to the saturated fat found in a double bacon cheeseburger and small fries. At home, it translates to the saturated fat found in 1 ounce of Swiss cheese, 1 tablespoon of butter, 1 chicken breast (without the skin), a handful of almonds, 2 eggs, 2 tablespoons of ranch salad dressing, and a quarter-pound hamburger. By the way, note how much more you can eat at home. (You'll learn more details in Week 3.)

Sources of Trans Fats	Healthier Alternatives
Creamy, commercially prepared salad dressings	Olive oil/vinegar, Enova oil, walnut oil
Fast-food fries, frozen fries	Pretzels, air-popped popcorn, whole wheat matzo and crackers
Frozen entrées, fried fast foods	Frozen, unprocessed meat; poultry; fish; rice; and vegetables*
Stick margarine	Tub margarine
Frosting	Glazes or fruit purees, candy, meringues, peppermints, dried fruit

*Not breaded or fried; prepared without sauces made with partially hydrogenated oils, which have trans fats

- **Trans-fatty acids.** Listed on food ingredient labels as partially hydrogenated and hydrogenated oils, these fats are often found in snack foods, baked goods, frozen breaded entrées, and commercially prepared salad dressings, among other products. **Advice:** Keep trans fats as low as possible, preferably less than 1 percent of total calories, because they, too, increase levels of LDL. Revised food labels make it easier to determine if a food contains trans fats, which are considered more dangerous than saturated fats in raising heart disease risk. Some products list zero trans fats on the nutrition facts label and then include partially hydrogenated or hydrogenated fats in the ingredients label. **The secret is that if a product contains less than half a gram of trans fats per serving, it can state that is has zero trans fats.** Also, deodorization of some healthy oils produces trace amounts of trans fats. If the label says zero, consider that

HOW TO USE THE NUTRITION FACTS LABEL

Nutrition Facts

Start here ———▶ Serving Size 1 cup (228g)
Servings Per Container 2

Amount Per Serving

Check calories **Calories** 250   Calories from Fat 110

% Daily Value*

Total Fat 12g	**18%**
Saturated Fat 3g	**15%**
Trans Fat 3g	
Cholesterol 30mg	**10%**
Sodium 470mg	**20%**
Potassium 700mg	**20%**
Total Carbohydrate 31g	**10%**
Dietary Fiber 0g	**0%**
Sugars 5g	
Protein 5g	

Limit these
nutrients

Vitamin A	4%
Vitamin C	2%
Calcium	20%
Iron	4%

Get enough of
these nutrients

* Percent Daily Values are based on a 2,000 calorie diet.
Your Daily Values may be higher or lower depending on
your calorie needs.

	Calories:	2,000	2,500
Total Fat	Less than	65g	80g
Sat Fat	Less than	20g	25g
Cholesterol	Less than	300mg	300mg
Sodium	Less than	2,400mg	2,400mg
Total Carbohydrate		300g	375g
Dietary Fiber		25g	30g

Footnote

Quick Guide to Percent Daily Value

• 5% or less is low

• 20% or more is high

the food either has no trans fat or very low amounts, even if the ingredients label lists partially hydrogenated fat.

- **Cholesterol**. Leading sources include egg yolks, liver and other organ meats, and full-fat dairy products. **Advice:** Limit to 300 milligrams per day—about the amount found in one egg yolk—since cholesterol can also hike low-density lipoprotein, a damaging form of blood cholesterol. Limit to three to four egg yolks per week if you already have heart disease.

Smart Choices

No need to mourn the reduction of saturated fat, trans fats, or cholesterol. There are plenty of healthy fats to add to your daily diet and there's international scientific consensus that doing so is very wise.

Healthy fats not only help reduce the risk of heart disease, there's also growing evidence that they may preserve brain power, keep joints protected from arthritis, and even improve mood. Plus, healthy fat comes in tantalizing foods from avocados and nuts to seafood. So the secret of a healthy diet is to reach for these healthy fats, which provide mono- and polyunsaturated fat. No need to bore you with all the details, but suffice it to say that it's the chemical bonds that make the difference between good and bad fats.

- **Avocados.** Creamy and delicious, avocados are about 80 percent fat, which might put them off-limits for some people. **The secret is that only 13 percent of those calories come from unhealthy saturated fat.** Although a quarter of an avocado has roughly 80 calories—about the same found in two pats of butter—it's loaded with vitamin E; potassium; the antioxidant lutein, which is good for the eyes, the skin, and the heart (and is now an ingredient in many multivitamins); plus healthy omega-3 fatty acids and other healthy fat.

- **Flaxseeds.** These tiny brown seeds are about half the size of sesame seeds and come packed with protein, fiber, and omega-3 fatty acids—a type of healthy fat that can't be manufactured by the body. Omega 3s are needed for proper growth and development of the brain and nervous system. They help lower blood cholesterol and blood pressure. They help prevent heart disease and stroke and may play a role in prevention of breast cancer. Flaxseeds can be ground with a coffee grinder or pepper mill onto salad, soup, cereal, or other foods. Or flaxseed oil can be used in salad dressings. Just don't use it for frying or sautéing, since flaxseed oil is quite unstable. Refrigerate both flaxseeds and flaxseed oil to give them a longer shelf life of about four months.

- **Nuts.** They're not only great for snacks; nuts contain enough protein to be an alternative to meat. Nuts also have complex carbs—less likely to spike blood sugar—a bit of fiber, vitamin E, and plenty of healthy fat. With nearly 200 calories per handful, however, they need to be eaten judiciously. In 2003, the Food and Drug Administration gave nuts a qualified health claim: "Evidence suggests, but does not prove, that eating one and a half ounces per day of most nuts as part of a diet low in saturated fat and cholesterol may reduce the risk of heart disease."

- **Olive and canola oil** are rich in monounsaturated fat. Replace butter and other saturated fat with these fats to help lower low-density lipoprotein (LDL), a dangerous form of blood cholesterol. Limited and still emerging scientific evidence suggests that eating about two tablespoons of olive oil daily may reduce the risk of coronary heart disease, according to the FDA. But be sure to use olive oil to replace a similar amount of saturated fat—not increase the total number of calories—you eat in a day.

- **Safflower oil, sunflower oil, soybean oil, tub margarine (without trans fats), and mayonnaise** contain healthy polyunsaturated fats. Substitute these oils for saturated fat, such as butter or lard, to help cut levels of LDL, one of the most damaging forms of cholesterol. But go easy, since too much polyunsaturated fat may cut levels of the protective form of blood cholesterol: high-density lipoprotein (HDL). Current expert guidelines from the federal government and the American Heart Association are to limit polyunsaturated fat calories to no more than 10 percent of total daily calories. That works out to about two tablespoons of tub margarine (without trans fats).

- **Healthy "margarines."** Take Control and Benecol are two margarinelike spreads that contain plant sterols and stanols—substances that help lower blood cholesterol levels as much as some cholesterol-lowering drugs. Use them in moderation (or choose their light versions), since they contain as many calories as regular margarine—about 45 calories per tablespoon—but none of the trans fats.

- **Seafood** is loaded with omega-3 fatty acids that are good for your heart, your brain, and your joints. There's even evidence to suggest that omega 3s may help guard against depression. Omega 3s lower the risk of a fatal irregular heartbeat. They improve the ratio of good cholesterol to bad in the blood, which cuts your odds of suffering a heart attack or stroke. And omega 3s help reduce inflammation, which has been linked to a host of ills, from arthritis to clogged arteries. The evidence is strong enough that the FDA granted a qualified health claim to omega-3 fatty acids. It notes that supportive but not conclusive research shows that consumption of two types of omega-3 fatty acids—EPA (eicosapentaenoic acid) and DHA (docosahexaenoic acid)—"may reduce the risk of coronary heart disease."

The Happy Fat?

That's what some scientists call omega-3 fatty acids because preliminary findings suggest they may help treat depression.

Omega-3 fatty acids include:

alpha-linolenic acid, which contains

- eicosapentaenoic acid (EPA)

Where to get it: soybean and canola oils, walnuts, flaxseeds

- docosahexaenoic acid (DHA)

Where to get it: fish and shellfish, especially salmon, tuna, trout

The FDA recommends that consumers not exceed 3 grams per day of EPA and DHA omega-3 fatty acids, with no more than 2 grams per day from a dietary supplement.

SOURCE: U.S. Food and Drug Administration

In 2000, the FDA announced a similar qualified health claim for dietary supplements containing the same types of omega-3 fatty acids. The agency advised that consumers not exceed more than a total of three grams per day of EPA and DHA omega-3 fatty acids and said that no more than two grams per day should come from a dietary supplement.

Advice: Eat two servings of seafood—about three to four ounces per serving—per week. Nearly all fish and seafood contains traces of mercury. For most people this doesn't pose a health problem, but for women of childbearing age and for children, eating some types of fish and seafood could be harmful. What to avoid? Shark, swordfish, king mackerel, and tilefish, according to both the Environmental Protection Agency and the FDA. What seafood is lowest in mercury? Shrimp, salmon, pollack, catfish, anchovies, and sardines.

And then there's tuna, one of the most popular types of fish. Canned light tuna is the tuna lowest in mercury, followed by "white" or albacore canned tuna and tuna steak. Federal experts caution women of childbearing age and children to limit consumption of tuna.

Tuna

Benefits: Pennies per serving, great taste, good source of protein and healthy omega-3 fatty acids.

Flavor tip: Buy tuna canned in olive oil. Drain excess oil; skip the mayonnaise.

Choose

- Light canned tuna, but women of childbearing age and children should not eat more than 12 ounces per week to avoid mercury contamination.

Limit

- No more than 6 ounces per week of fresh tuna steak or white or albacore canned tuna.

SOURCES: U.S. Food and Drug Administration; U.S. Environmental Protection Agency

---

FIBER

What if a couple of servings a day of food could help safeguard your health—and whittle your waistline? That's the simple—and surprising—power of fiber. It's the food that helps you feel full with just a few calories and is good enough at lowering cholesterol to earn a heart-healthy claim from the Food and Drug Administration.

Yet, like fruits and vegetables, fiber is overlooked and underconsumed—so much so that the 2005 Dietary Guidelines Advisory Committee put fiber on the list of shortfall nutrients that are "of concern" for adults and children.

So what gives fiber its muscle?

Beside keeping things "regular," fiber helps to thwart the development of both type 2 diabetes and heart disease. There's also tantalizing evidence that fiber may reduce the odds of developing colorectal cancer. Fiber seems to help with weight control. Women who consistently ate extra grams of fiber—about the amount found in a bowl of high-fiber cereal and a slice of whole wheat bread daily—had half the risk of obesity as those whose fiber intake gradually declined during a 12-year study. Not only did the high-fiber group eat about 150 fewer calories per day, but they had an eight-pound loss during the study. Compare that to a nearly 20-pound weight gain for those who skimped on fiber.

Men's waistlines can benefit from boosting fiber, too. A Harvard School of Public Health study found that those who ate just 12 grams more of fiber per day than other participants shrunk their belt size by half an inch over a decade.

How much fiber do you need? For women, about the amount found in a cup of beans and a couple of slices of whole wheat bread. For men, the amount found in a high-fiber cereal, a cup of beans, and a couple of slices of whole wheat bread—in short, about twice the fiber that most people consume. (If you want to know the exact numbers, it works out to 25 grams of fiber per day for most women; 38 grams for men. Adults 51 years and older need 21 grams per day for women; 30 grams for men.) You will learn more about how to boost fiber in Weeks 1, 2, and 5 of the Lean Plate Club Program.

Fiber
What the experts say:

19–50 years
   Women   25 grams/day
   Men   38 grams/day

51+
   Women   21 grams/day
   Men   30 grams/day

SOURCES: National Academy of Sciences Dietary Reference Intakes; 2005 Dietary Guidelines Advisory Committee Report

SUGAR

These days, you don't have to have a sweet tooth to wind up consuming a lot of added sugars without realizing it. Sugar is found in everything from ready-to-eat cereals and fruit juices to soft drinks, yogurt, and high-fiber whole wheat bread. Consumption of added sugars reached 147 pounds per person in 2001. Nearly half of that added sugar comes from high-fructose corn syrup, a trend that worries many nutrition experts. Some studies suggest that this sweet, thick syrup may help to undermine appetite control and possibly play a role in weight gain.

Both the National Academy of Sciences and the World Health Organization urge limiting intake of added sugars to between 10 to 25 percent of total calories. (On an average 2,000 calories per day, that works out to 200–500 calories—or about the amount found in a couple of brownies and a large scoop of Ben and Jerry's.)

Added Sugars

What the experts say: Limit to 10 to 25 percent of daily calories.

On 2,000 calories/day, that works out to 50 grams, or about that found in a 16-ounce soft drink.

SOURCES: World Health Organization; National Academy of Sciences, U.S. Department of Agriculture Nutrient Data Laboratory

---

In small amounts, added sugar isn't a villain, except, perhaps, for those worried about tooth decay. The problem is that added sugar, whether it is in table sugar, high-fructose corn syrup, honey, or any other sweet source, is dense in calories. Figure on 16 to 20 calories per teaspoon. It's also a nutritional lightweight, because it comes with no added minerals, vitamins, phytonutrients, fiber, or other key nutrients. Plus, foods high in added sugar tend to edge out healthier fare. So it's little wonder that the 2005 Dietary Guidelines Committee found that those who eat large amounts of food and beverages high in added sugars "tend to consume more calories but smaller amounts of micronutrients." Current U.S. dietary recommendations echo the advice of the World Health Organization. Simply put, eat a diet low in added sugars. Translated to food, that means

---

Here's the Secret to Soothe a Sweet Tooth

If you're craving a candy bar, cookie, or some other sugary treat a couple of hours after lunch, you may not be eating enough at your midday meal. Try adding 100 healthy calories to lunch. Or plan a healthy snack (about 100–200 calories) *before* your sweet tooth strikes.

Possible choices: Nonfat plain yogurt with fruit or a dab of honey; ready-to-eat whole-grain cereal with skim milk; dried fruit mixture and nuts; honey-roasted soybeans or nuts; hot cocoa made with skim milk; fruit with a teaspoon of peanut butter; snack bar, such as Pria, Kashi, Luna, Special K, or Health Valley.

---

soothing your sweet tooth with fruit wherever possible. It means choosing unsweetened cereals over sugar-coated varieties and opting for soft drinks, coffee, and tea that are lightly sweetened with sugar or are sweetened with sugar substitutes instead of sugar. And it means saving the usual sugary suspects—cookies, pies, cakes, and candy—for very special occasions.

Sugar Substitutes

If you're craving something sweet and don't want to consume added calories, food and drink sweetened with sugar substitutes are options. A number of Lean Plate Club members cook with Splenda, one of the newer sugar substitutes on the market, with good results. But just because a food contains a sugar substitute doesn't mean that it's automatically low in calories. For example, ice cream and other frozen desserts sweetened with sugar substitutes can still have as many calories as the regular stuff because they contain the same—or more—fat. Here's a brief guide to the most widely used sugar substitutes.

- **Acesulfame K.** Sold as Sunnett, Acesulfame K is not metabolized by the body and so contains zero calories. Discovered in 1967, Acesulfame K was first approved by the FDA in 1988 and now is used in a wide variety of foods and beverages, from baked goods to diet soft drinks. This sugar substitute is about 200 times sweeter than sugar and does not break down when cooked or baked—one reason why it's now found in more than 4,000 different products.

- **Aspartame.** Best known as NutraSweet and Equal, aspartame is used in more than 6,000 products by more than 200 million people worldwide. It was approved as a "tabletop" sweetener by the Food and Drug Administration in 1981. Since then it's been approved for use in various foods and beverages by the FDA. It contains two amino acids—building blocks of protein—and methanol, an alcohol. Drawback: Aspartame loses sweetness under heat, so it's not good for baking or cooking. One developing concern: In 2005, the Center for Science in the Public Interest, a consumer advocacy group, asked the FDA to request new animal studies of aspartame at the government's National Toxicology Program after a long-term study by Italian researchers found a statistically signficiant increase in lymphomas and leukemias among female rats given aspartame. While rats obviously aren't the same as people, CSPI suggested that consumers and food manufacturers switch to sucralose (Splenda) until more tests can be done—yet another reason to eat a varied diet, moderate in all things.

- **Neotame.** Approved in 2002 by the FDA, Neotame contains zero calories and is at least 7,000 times sweeter than sugar. It's made from two amino acids and is approved for use in a wide variety of products, from sugarless chewing gum to frozen desserts, and as a "tabletop" sweetener. Neotame holds up well under high temperatures, so it can be used in cooking and baking.

To learn more on sugar substitutes, log on to the Food and Drug Administration Web site, www.fda.gov.

Or check out the Calorie Control Council, a nonprofit group funded in part by the food industry, at www.caloriecontrolcouncil.org/lowcal.html.

- **Saccharin.** Known commercially as Sweet'N Low, saccharin has been sold for more than a century. In 1977, a Canadian study found that saccharin caused bladder cancer in rats. The FDA considered banning saccharin, but Congress passed a bill to give saccharin a reprieve and has extended the moratorium on banning it several times since then. Saccharin is used in diet soft drinks, as a sweetener in place of table sugar, and in cooking and baking since it is stable at high temperatures.

- **Sucralose.** Sold as Splenda, sucraclose is made from sugar that has three chlorine atoms added to it. British researchers first discovered sucralose in 1976. It was approved by the FDA in 1999 and is now used in more than 80 countries in foods and beverages and as a "tabletop" sweetener.

- **Sugar alcohols.** You'll find them listed as xylitol, sorbitol, mannitol, and malitol in a wide variety of products, from chewing gum to energy bars. Not technically sugar substitutes, sugar alcohols are nonetheless slightly lower in calories than sugar. Because they don't spike blood sugar levels the way sugar does, sugar alcohols are often used in foods for people with diabetes. They also don't appear to cause tooth decay. But they can cause some gastrointestinal distress, including loose bowels in some people, especially when eaten in large quantities.

THE SALT OF THE EARTH

Don't forget about another food ingredient: sodium. According to the National Academy of Sciences, 95 percent of men and 75 percent of women eat too much salt.

Removing the saltshaker from the table is a noble step, but will do only a little to cut sodium intake. That's because up to 80 percent of the sodium consumed these days comes from processed food and restaurant fare. And it's not just the usual suspects—french fries, olives, pickles, potato chips, canned soup, or tomato sauce—that are the leading culprits. A 2005 survey by the Center for Science in the Public Interest found that bread is the number one source of sodium in the American diet. CSPI estimates that the rise in salt consumption over the last 30 years has led to 150,000 premature deaths annually, most of them related to high blood pressure and its complications.

Advice: The lower the better for sodium. Limit intake to 2,300 milligrams if you're 45 years or younger. That's equal to about a teaspoon of salt. If you're age 45 to 70, aim for 1,500 milligrams per day or less. That's also the guideline for African Americans, because of a higher risk for high blood pressure, and for those of any age who have been diagnosed with elevated blood pressure, and a good idea for everyone who doesn't want to see blood pressure rise with age. Those over 70 years need 1,200 milligrams per day or less, according to the National Academy of Sciences.

Warning: Counting sodium grams can be tedious. Read the nutrition facts labels on products. Products that contain 5 percent or less of the daily value are considered low in sodium; those that have 20 percent or more are considered high in sodium. Anything in between is considered moderate in sodium. Remember that it's not one meal—or one day—of high sodium that counts but the trend over time.

Here's a secret: Eat more foods high in potassium to help counterbalance the effects of a high-sodium diet, according to findings of the federally funded DASH (Dietary Approaches to Stop Hypertension). Fruits and vegetables are prime sources of potassium. Learn more in Week 1 of the Lean Plate Club Program. Also look for assistance from some food companies, which are voluntarily adding potassium to the nutrition facts labels.

WATER

"Drink eight to ten glasses of water daily" used to be the kind of commonsense advice that ranked with "Brush your teeth three times daily" and "Look twice before crossing the street." In 2004, an expert panel convened by the National Academy of Sciences concluded that thirst—not drinking a set number of glasses of water—is the best guide for proper hydration.

The academy also broke new ground in concluding that all beverages—yes, even coffee, tea, juice, diet or regular sodas, and alcohol—contribute toward meeting the daily fluid intake. For most men, that works out to about 13 cups daily. For most women, about nine cups.

In the past, experts advised not including caffeinated or alcoholic drinks in the daily mix, because they can act as diuretics and cause water loss. The academy has concluded that for most adults, this water loss is transient and not significant. Besides water—whether sparkling, flavored with fruit or vitamins, or just plain—and other beverages, water-filled foods, including soups and stews and fruits and vegetables, provide additional ways to help hydrate the body and quench thirst, still the best guide to how much to drink.

ALCOHOL

A little bit of alcohol with meals may be good for your heart, but often lost in the translation from scientific finding to uncorking a bottle of spirits, wine, or brew are the caveats and health downsides. Did you know, for example, that the protective effects of alcohol for the heart apply only to men over 40 and women past menopause? Or that the health benefits of drinking alcohol peak at one drink per day for women, two drinks daily for men? Aside from the well-known potential for abuse and addiction, there are a number of nutritional downsides to alcohol. A gram of alcohol has 7 calories, nearly double that of protein or carbs. Plus, alcohol is so easily metabolized that it is more likely than either protein or carbs to be stored directly as fat—a fact to take into consideration the next time you're tempted to split of bottle of wine with a friend.

One "drink" equals

- 5-ounce glass of wine
- 2½ ounces of port, sherry, or dessert wine
- 12 ounces of beer (lite, regular, or low-carb)
- 1½ ounces of 80-proof distilled spirits

SOURCES: 2005 U.S. Dietary Guidelines; Wine Institute

For women, imbibing raises some special health concerns, especially for breast cancer. Each ounce of alcohol increases the risk of developing breast cancer. During pregnancy and while trying to conceive, teetotalling is the only safe option for the fetus. When you toast, remember this: Potential health benefits come only from light to moderate consumption of alcohol—at most, one drink daily for women, two per day for men, which is best consumed with meals rather than as cocktails before them to slow alcohol absorption.

Here's the secret: Skip the cocktails. Imbibe only at meals to help slow absorption of alcohol.

If you skip drinking alcohol during the week, that doesn't mean that you can make up for it by bingeing with extra rounds on the weekends. The recommended amount is a use-it-or-lose-it daily limit.

Here's the secret: Use a 1-ounce aperitif glass to stretch a 5-ounce glass of wine into 5 sipping servings to slow consumption. You may find you're satisfied after only 1 or 2, which halves the calories and the alcohol.

Five

GET PHYSICAL

Stand up. Reach for the ceiling. Let your arms and fingertips stretch as far as they will comfortably go. Take a deep breath and slowly exhale as you lower your arms. Feel a brief moment of both relaxation and energy? That's just a taste of what most people miss these days by being way too inactive.

"Chronically sedentary" describes the majority of adults as well as many kids and teens. Even those who make regular trips to the gym remain inactive for the remainder of the day. Modern conveniences from computers to remote controls, power windows, and even electric toothbrushes are slowly but surely eliminating physical activity from our lives.

Think about it. When was the last time you hoofed it to a colleague's office to ask a question instead of sending an e-mail? When did you open a can with a hand-cranked opener instead of an electric one? When did you take the stairs instead of waiting in line to ride the escalator or elevator? When did you stand up and change the channel manually on the television instead of using the remote control?

Even when people try to get more activity, they're often stymied. Locked staircases prevent walking from floor to floor in many buildings. Housing developments are increasingly designed without sidewalks. Urban planners have made crossing the street in many major cities a dangerous and uninviting activity. Even some golf courses, which used to encourage walking the links, now require players to ride in electric carts to keep them moving quickly from hole to hole.

One of the biggest impediments to regular exercise is time.

"What's the best physical activity I can do?" is the question that I often get asked by Lean Plate Club members. The answer is simple: The best physical activity is the one that you do regularly. It doesn't matter whether it's ballroom dancing or tae bo. To be successful at getting fitter and leaner, you need to find ways to make physical activity as much a part of your daily routine as brushing your teeth. My guess is that you wouldn't consider not doing that!

The importance of physical activity goes way beyond the desire to fit into a smaller suit, a slim pair of jeans, or a bikini. Decades of research show unequivocally that regular physical activity is one of the best things that you do for your health, regardless of your age, your weight, your gender, or your present physical limitations. There is no time of life when you can't reap the benefits of physical activity. In fact, the latest research suggests that most of the physical changes chalked up to growing old—insulin resistance, decreased lung capacity, muscle loss, and elevated blood pressure—are due mostly to inactivity. By moving more, you can not only help prevent these problems but also reverse some of them.

Regular, moderate physical activity also improves mental functioning, sleep, and energy. It boosts mood, cuts the risk of depression, helps control anxiety, and reduces stress. And, likely of most interest to you, physical activity helps control, combat, and trim unwanted pounds.

Where many people go wrong is in overestimating the number of calories burned with physical activity. "Sally, I don't understand. I've been walking a mile a day for the past two weeks, and I've only lost a pound" is the kind of message I frequently field on Lean Plate Club Web chats and in e-mails. "Why am I not losing more weight?"

WHAT'S MODERATE PHYSICAL ACTIVITY?

	Calories/Hour*
Hiking	367
Light gardening/yard work	331
Dancing	331
Golfing (walk/carry clubs)	331
Biking (< 10 mph)	294
Walking (3.5 mph, 17 min/mi)	279
Weight lifting	220

SOURCE: 2005 U.S. Dietary Guidelines

*Based on a 154-pound person

Here's the secret: While exercise helps to boost metabolism, it doesn't boost it a lot. So a 150-pound person who walks a mile in 15 minutes burns about 85 calories—less than the amount found in a small chocolate chip cookie and about half the number of calories found in a small bag of potato chips. Walk 15 minutes daily for a week, and you chalk up 595 calories. Since it takes a deficit of 3,500 calories to lose a pound, those daily 15-minute walks help trim only about a sixth of a pound per week. That's much less than most people expect and it's why the public health officials urge us to aim for at least 30 minutes daily to reduce the risk of chronic diseases and improve fitness.

By the way, 30 minutes is in addition to the usual activities that you do at home and work.

Losing weight requires more physical activity. How much more? At least 60 minutes of moderate daily activity and maybe up to 90 minutes, for weight loss. (Walking at a brisk 4-mph pace—about 15 minutes per mile—is considered a moderate activity.)

Move It!

Minimum daily: 30 minutes of moderate activity, such as brisk walking. (This is in addition to regular daily work or home activities.)

Alternative: 20 minutes of vigorous activity (such as jogging) three times weekly.

To lose weight: 60 minutes/day of moderate to vigorous activity.

To maintain weight loss (or prevent weight gain with age): 60 to 90 minutes daily of moderate activity.

Plus:

To build/maintain muscle: Resistance training (weight lifting, resistance elastic bands, calisthenics) two or more times per week to condition major muscles.

To maintain flexibility: Stretching exercises at least three times per week.

SOURCES: 2005 Dietary Guidelines Advisory Committee; American Council on Exercise; American College of Sports Medicine.

Why doubling or tripling activity is necessary to successfully shed pounds and keep it off is still not understood. Exercise physiologists believe that yo-yo dieting may be to blame. Much of the evidence comes from the National Weight Control Registry, a group of several thousand "successful losers" who have shed an average of 60 pounds and kept it off for an average of five years.

Each time you lose weight, you shed lean muscle along with the fat. That results in a higher percentage of body fat with repeated weight cycling. Since fat burns fewer calories than muscle, as muscle mass declines, it takes more activity to burn the same number of calories. That's another reason why it's important to reach a healthy weight and stay there for good.

WHAT'S VIGOROUS PHYSICAL ACTIVITY?

	Calories/Hour*
Running/jogging (5 mph)	588
Biking (> 10 mph)	588
Swimming (slow freestyle laps)	514
Aerobics	478
Walking (4.5 mph)	464
Heavy yard work (chopping wood)	441
Basketball (intensive)	441
Weight training (intensive)	441

SOURCE: 2005 U.S. Dietary Guidelines

*Based on a 154-pound person

Sixty to 90 minutes can sound daunting, especially to the chronically sedentary. Before you throw in the towel, **here's a secret you need to know: You don't have to do this activity all at one time.** In fact, there's plenty of evidence from the University of Virginia, the University of Pittsburgh, the University of Ulster, Brown University, and other well-regarded medical institutions that short bouts of exercise—as little as ten minutes at a time—are just as effective as longer, sustained workouts to trim pounds or boost fitness. During the eight-week Lean Plate Club Program, you'll also learn how "lifestyle activities"—hoofing it on errands, taking the stairs, getting off the bus or metro a stop early and walking the rest of the distance—are just as effective as regular, organized exercise in burning more calories.

Muscle Beach

Amount of muscles built by average person with weight training: 4 pounds.

Time required to build muscle: at least 6 weeks with workouts three times per week.

Calories burned per pound of lean muscle: 35–40 per day.

Calories burned per pound of fat: 2–3 per day.

SOURCES: American Council on Exercise; William Kraemer, Ph.D., University of Connecticut Human Performance Laboratory

---

Weight training can also help move the bathroom scale in your favor. Lifting free weights or working out with weight machines are the obvious, traditional ways of building muscle. But there are plenty of other activities to help strengthen and tone muscles. You'll learn that and more in the Lean Plate Club Program, including "executive sit-ups" and other secret exercises that help preserve posture, protect the back, and reduce injury elsewhere in the body.

Part Two

THE LEAN PLATE CLUB EIGHT-WEEK PROGRAM

OVERVIEW: WHAT YOU CAN *ADD* TO YOUR LIFE

The Lean Plate Club column, Web chat, and newsletter have helped millions of members eat smart and move more as they work to achieve a healthier weight. By taking the eight-week Lean Plate Club challenge, you'll be joining them in adding healthy food and physical activity to your life.

During the next eight weeks, you'll learn how to:

- Eat smart by choosing the healthiest foods that you like best. You'll find lists to help guide you with grocery shopping, eating out, and cooking at home.

- Move more by finding the physical activities you enjoy most. It's a simple fact: If you don't like an activity, you likely won't stick with it. Weekly goals will help you gradually get more active every day, finding the activities that you enjoy most and the workout routines that add exercise to your daily life.

- Set reasonable goals. It's the best way to achieve long-lasting habits. Here's a brief summary of what you can expect during the next eight weeks:

Week 1: What Colors Are in Your Rainbow?

Start with the basics: Add fruits and vegetables. Find them hard to swallow? No problem. You'll learn the secret of eating hidden fruit and vegetables so that even the most committed fruits and vegetable haters can find something to savor. You'll also find resources to help you with recipes and menus.

All Sizes Fit: No need to work up a sweat. Don't change a thing. Just track how much physical activity you get right now. And buy a pedometer. Find out how best to wear it on page 140.

Week 2: Fiber Up!

It used to be called roughage. Today it's known as fiber. No matter what its name, Americans still don't eat enough. Don't worry, chewing hay is not required. There are plenty of other healthy, great-tasting fibers to add to your daily life. And the bonus: You will feel fuller with fewer calories. You'll also find easy ways to incorporate more fiber plus recipes to help you do it. And of course, there is always inspiration from other Lean Plate Club members to help you.

All Sizes Fit: Easy. Simply add a two-minute walk daily. Everyone—yes, even you!—can do that. And if you're already a dedicated gymgoer, you'll learn why you still can use some extra daily activity.

Week 3: Swap the Bad for the Good

Discover the secret of smart substitutions—you know, eliminating unhealthy fats and replacing them with the good stuff: avocados, olives, nuts, and more. In moderation, of course. Learn what oils to choose and find some healthy, great-tasting recipes to put your new habits into practice.

All Sizes Fit: Add five more minutes to your daily walk—enough to splurge on a tablespoon of whipped cream on top of your sliced fruit and slivered nuts.

Week 4: Protein Power

This week's secret: Add protein to help you feel full and rev your metabolism—a little. Learn how much to add and what types of protein are the smartest choices, including a special section for vegetarians and vegans.

All Sizes Fit: Boost physical activity to ten minutes daily—one-third of the way toward the recommended goal. And yes, it's okay to do more, as long as you're consistent with the ten minutes daily.

Week 5: Clean Up Your Carbs

Whole grains are the secret ingredients this week. You need three servings daily to meet the latest recommendations for healthful nutrition. You'll learn the smartest ways to meet that goal, with special tips for those following lower-carb approaches.

All Sizes Fit: Keep the ten-minute daily walk, add resistance training three times weekly to start building muscle—a great way to help rev your metabolism.

Week 6: Count on Calcium

You already know that calcium is good for your bones. It also helps the heart and it may be good for other parts of the body, too. You'll learn how to meet the three recommended servings daily and why vitamin D is an important ally in this effort. Special help for those with lactose intolerance, vegetarians, and vegans.

All Sizes Fit: Boost daily activity to 20 minutes—two-thirds of the way to the recommended amount—and keep doing that resistance training.

Week 7: Mindful Eating

Learn the secret of avoiding nutritional mischief. Discover how to tame your trigger foods, banish nighttime eating, and evade more habits that can undermine your healthier habits.

All Sizes Fit: Add five more minutes of daily activity for a total of 25 minutes, boost the weights lifted, and begin stretching to increase your flexibility.

Week 8: Sleep to Reach Your Dreams

Discover why it's a bad idea to burn the candle at both ends. Learn how eight hours of z's nightly can be your secret weapon for improving a variety of measures, from better blood sugar levels to evening out insulin secretion and other hormone levels—all important to help you achieve a healthier weight.

All Sizes Fit: Add five more minutes daily to your activity level and you've met the basic requirement for 30 minutes daily of physical activity. That's an important habit to help you stay at a healthy weight for life.

Six

WEEK 1: WHAT COLORS ARE IN YOUR RAINBOW?

My vegetable love should grow, vaster than empires and more slow.

—Andrew Marvell, 1621–1678

A melon for ecstasy!

—Middle Eastern adage

You already know the obvious: Fruits and vegetables are good for your health. The more you eat, the better. This is one of the food groups where it's okay to go wild. In fact, go really, really wild. Eating fruit is a great way to soothe an afternoon sweet tooth and it's hard to find better-tasting snacks—with more crunch and fewer calories—than a platter of vegetables and some salsa or guacamole for dipping.

Is your mouth watering yet?

If the idea of boosting fruits and vegetables still seems daunting, you're not alone. Many Lean Plate Club members report being skeptical, too—until they try it. As one LPC member noted during a Web chat, "Three years ago I was 40-plus pounds heavier and wouldn't touch a vegetable or fruit with a ten-foot pole. I was pretty miserable and could barely make it up the stairs without gasping for breath. I decided one day to make life changes (I never say diet!) and gradually added fitness and healthy eating to my life. I can tell you that I feel so much better. I now love fruit and vegetables—all sorts of colors. I love to make fruit smoothies for breakfast and for dinner, I grill red, green, and yellow peppers with onions and squash. I eat these with some brown rice and salsa. Very delicious!"

The secret is this: It's a whole lot easier than you think to eat the recommended servings daily, in part because the serving sizes are smaller than you may imagine. Making fruits and vegetables a priority not only can help you reach a healthier weight but also can keep you out of nutritional mischief. Learn to reach first for fruits and vegetables when you're hungry, and you'll discover how full they help you feel. As this Lean Plate Club member notes, "I now swear by the two-pound bag of baby carrots that I buy weekly. I'm usually starving when I get home but won't be eating for at least another 45 minutes. I throw some baby carrots and water into the microwave and steam those babies for a few minutes. I spray them with I Can't Believe It's Not Butter and I'm good to go. Not only do I sneak in some healthy veggies but (much more importantly) I'm far less likely to tear into my husband's stash of baked Doritos!"

COLOR YOUR PLATE

Keep in mind two simple tips as you add more fruits and vegetables this week:

- Go for variety. It's as important as quantity in reaping all the nutritional benefits from fruits and vegetables.

- Fresh produce is fine, but frozen, canned, and dried provide similar nutritional benefits. They can help you stretch food dollars and allow you to have fruits and vegetables always on hand.

Consult the table below to find out the minimum number of servings of fruits and vegetables you need to consume daily. And go ahead, add more if you want, provided that they're not deep-fat fried or loaded with added sugar. Since fruits and vegetables come with fiber and water, they'll help you feel full on fewer calories than many other foods.

ADD FRUITS AND VEGETABLES ACCORDING TO YOUR DAILY CALORIE NEEDS

This table shows the minimum needed. More servings are okay.

Daily calories	Fruit (cups)	Vegetables (cups)
1,000	1	1
1,200	1	1½
1,400	1½	1½
1,600	1½	2
1,800	1½	2½
2,000	2	2½
2,400	2	3
2,600	2	3½
2,800	2½	3½
3,000	2½	4
3,200	2½	4

SOURCE: 2005 U.S. Dietary Guidelines

Hungry? Reach into the Cookie Jar

Find or purchase an empty cookie jar and place it on your kitchen counter. When you have a few minutes, cut up strips of paper. On each strip, write something that you could do when you feel hungry. Some examples:

1. Clean out a drawer.
2. Sweep the front walk.
3. Read a book for five minutes.
4. Take a walk around the block.
5. Brush or floss your teeth.
6. Polish a piece of silver.
7. Go after the cobwebs in the corners.
8. Mend a piece of clothing.
9. Do ten push-ups.
10. Walk in place for five minutes.
11. Write a letter to a friend.
12. Call a relative you haven't talked to in a very long time.
13. Wash a window or a mirror.
14. Spend five minutes organizing your CDs or iPod.
15. Rearrange your medicine chest.
16. Put five pictures in an album.
17. Knit or crochet for a few minutes.
18. Soak in the tub.
19. Give yourself a manicure.
20. Brush your dog or pet your cat.

You get the idea. Imagination is your only limitation. When you feel hungry—and you know that it's not real hunger that you're experiencing—reach into the cookie jar. Pull out a strip. Do whatever activity you pull out.

What's in a Cup?

Forget the vague "servings" that were a hallmark of past dietary guidelines. Nutrition experts have wised up and use the common measurements found in every kitchen.

Here's the simple conversion for calculating 1 cup of fruit and vegetables.

Fruit

1 cup = 1 piece of fruit

       = 1 cup juice (preferably without added sugar)

       = ½ cup dried fruit

Vegetables

1 cup = 1 cup of raw or cooked vegetables

       = 1 cup of vegetable juice

       = 2 cups of raw leafy greens, such as fresh spinach, lettuce, arugula

For more specifics, see the charts on pages 128–29 and 133–36.

SOURCES: USDA www.MyPyramid.gov; 2005 U.S. Dietary Guidelines

---

Here's the secret: Fruits and vegetables add flavor, texture, and variety, and provide literally thousands of beneficial phytonutrients. Phytonutrients are healthful substances that come from plants. Scientists are still sorting out all their actions in the body, but they appear to help account for food synergy—beneficial chemical reactions that seem to occur from food. For now, researchers have been unable to duplicate these helpful effects with dietary supplements.

To help you paint your daily menu like an artist, photocopy the following lists, which are arranged by color and fruit/vegetable

---

Note to Low-Carb or Healthy Carb Followers

Nonstarchy, green vegetables are among the lowest in carbs. Boost these to keep closer to recommended intake levels on early phases of South Beach and Atkins and to provide additional fiber, since fruit is not allowed.

---

category. Check your favorites from each group and take this list grocery shopping. If you need more motivation to boost fruit and vegetable intake this week, read the fine print for some of the additional health benefits that come from consuming a diet rich in fruits and veggies.

Note to Glycemic Index Followers*

- **Fruits** Apples, blackberries, blueberries, raspberries, strawberries, kiwi, grapes, grapefruit, oranges, pears, and plums are among the lower glycemic index fruit.
- **Vegetables** Asparagus, broccoli, greens (of all types), cauliflower, carrots, celery, cucumbers, leeks, lettuce, mushrooms, peppers, okra, spinach, and tomatoes are among the lower glycemic index vegetables.
- **Potatoes** If you're hankering for a potato, make it small and sweet, purple or red, to stay lower on the glycemic index. Top it with some low-fat yogurt, nonfat sour cream, a little low-fat cheese, or some veggies. The protein and fiber in these foods will help lower the potato's glycemic index.

*The U.S. Dietary Guidelines Scientific Advisory Committee reviewed the glycemic index studies and concluded that at the present time there is still insufficient evidence to base food choices on the glycemic index.

Ann Arbor, Mich.: Hi, Sally. We were calling out way too much for Chinese food until I started buying the frozen, ready-for-stir-frying veggies. With a low-fat bottled stir-fry sauce (though we usually make our own), it's an inexpensive, quick, healthy dinner.

Reach for Red and Deep Pink

Among the key ingredients: Vitamin C, anthocyanins, and lycopene, a substance that appears to reduce the risk of certain cancers, including prostate cancer.

Fruits
Apples
Blood oranges
Cactus pears
Cherries
Cranberries
Guava
Pink grapefruit
Pomegranates
Raspberries
Strawberries
Watermelon

Vegetables
Beets
Kidney beans
Radicchio
Radishes
Red beans
Red cabbage
Red lentils

Red onions
Red peppers
Tamarillos
Tomatoes
Tomato juice
V8 juice

Go Green

Among the key ingredients: Carotenoids including lutein and zexanthin that act like antioxidants, gobbling up damaging free radicals—substances linked to cancer and aging. Antioxidants also help preserve vision by protecting the retina.

Fruits
Avocado
Cherimoya
Green apples (Granny Smith and others)
Green grapes
Honeydew melon
Kiwi
Limes
Pears

Vegetables
Artichokes
Arugula
Asparagus
Broccoli*
Broccoli rabe
Brussels sprouts*
Cabbage*
Cactus pads

Cauliflower*
Celery
Chayote squash
Chinese cabbage (napa/bok choy)*
Chinese long beans
Chipotle chilies
Collards
Cucumbers
Edamame
Endive
Escarole
Fennel
Green beans
Green onions
Green peppers
Kale
Kohlrabi (leaves)
Leeks
Lettuce (all varieties)
Mustard greens
Okra
Poblano chilies
Rapini
Snap peas
Snow peas
Spinach
Tomatillos
Turnips*
Zucchini

---

*Cruciferous vegetables that help prevent cancer. Eat several times per week.

Mellow Yellow and Orange

Among the key ingredients: Beta-carotene, which is converted in the body to vitamin A. It boosts immunity and protects vision. Also vitamins C and E, as well as folate—a B vitamin that helps prevent some serious birth defects, such as spina bifida. Pineapple also has a natural enzyme—bromelain—that aids in digestion and reduces bloating.

Fruits
Apricots
Asian pears
Bananas
Cantaloupe
Clementines
Golden delicious apples
Grapefruit
Kiwano/horned melon
Kumquats
Lemons
Mandarin oranges
Mangoes
Nectarines
Oranges
Orange juice
Papayas
Peaches
Pepino melon
Pineapple
Plantains
Quince
Star fruit

Tangerines
Yellow raisins

Vegetables
Butternut squash
Carrots
Corn
Golden nugget squash
Pumpkin
Rutabagas
Spaghetti squash
Summer squash
Sweet dumpling squash
Sweet potatoes

Get the Blues and Go Purple

Among the key ingredients: health-giving flavonoids and antho-cyanins that may help defend against cancer-causing agents, known as carcinogens. Also often rich in vitamin C, folate, fiber, and potassium, important for controlling blood pressure and heart function.

Fruits
Blackberries
Blueberries
Elderberries
Passion fruit
Plums
Dried plums (prunes)
Purple grapes
Raisins

Vegetables
Blue corn
Eggplant
Purple asparagus
Purple cabbage
Purple new potatoes

Win with White

Among the key ingredients: allicin, which reduces blood pressure and cholesterol and increases immunity.

Fruits
Bananas
Manzano bananas
Lychees
Pears
Plantains

Vegetables
Cauliflower
Daikon
Fennel
Garlic
Jicama
Kohlrabi (bulbs)
Leeks
Malanga
Mushrooms
Onions
Parsnips

Potatoes
Scallions
Shallots
Sunchokes
Turnips
Water chestnuts

HOW TO EAT MORE FRUITS AND VEGETABLES

Now that you know what to eat, here are some secrets to add more fruit and vegetables to your plate.

Add a fruit or vegetable to every meal and snack. That will go a long way toward meeting the daily goal. So top your breakfast cereal with raisins, have a banana with your midmorning coffee, and order a fruit cup for dessert at lunch. At dinner, make half your plate vegetables.

Look for hidden vegetable and fruit sources. Think hummus, baba ghanoush, guacamole, salsa, and bean dip. Boost the vegetable quotient even higher by using slices of red, yellow, or green peppers, celery stalks, and other vegetables to dip into them, rather than potato or corn chips that are higher in calories and fat. Other smart dipping choices: baby carrots, broccoli florets, and zucchini spears. A half cup of dip is about equal to one-half to one serving of vegetables, depending on how it's made.

PUT IT INTO PRACTICE
WHAT COUNTS AS 1 CUP OF FRUIT?

One cup of fruit or 100% fruit juice, or ½ cup of dried fruit, generally equals 1 cup from the fruit group. The following specific amounts count as 1 cup of fruit (in some cases equivalents for ½ cup are also shown) toward your daily recommended intake.

	Amount that counts as 1 cup	Amount that counts as ½ cup
Apple	½ large (3¼" diameter)	
	1 small (2½" diameter)	
	1 cup sliced or chopped, raw or cooked	½ cup sliced or chopped, raw or cooked
Applesauce	1 cup	1 snack container (4 ounces)
Banana	1 cup sliced	1 small (less than 6" long)
	1 large (8"–9" long)	
Cantaloupe	1 cup diced or melon balls	1 medium wedge (⅛ of a medium melon)
Grapefruit	1 medium (4" diameter)	½ medium (4" diameter)
	1 cup sections	
Grapes	1 cup whole or cut up	
	32 seedless	16 seedless
Mixed fruit (fruit cocktail)	1 cup diced or sliced, raw or canned, drained	1 snack container (4 ounces) drained
Orange	1 large (3" diameter)	1 small (2½" diameter)
	1 cup sections	
Orange, mandarin	1 cup canned, drained	
Peach	1 large (3" diameter)	1 small (2" diameter)
	1 cup sliced or diced, raw, cooked, or canned, drained	1 snack container (4 ounces) drained

	Amount that counts as 1 cup	Amount that counts as ½ cup
	2 halves, canned	
Pear	1 medium (6 ounces)	1 snack container (4 ounces) drained
	1 cup sliced or diced, raw, cooked, or canned, drained	
Pineapple	1 cup chunks, sliced or crushed, raw, cooked, or canned, drained	1 snack container (4 ounces) drained
Plum	1 cup sliced, raw or cooked	
	3 medium or 2 large	1 large
Strawberries	about 8 large	
	1 cup whole, halved, or sliced, fresh or frozen	½ cup whole, halved, or sliced
Watermelon	1 small wedge (1" thick)	6 balls
	1 cup diced or balls	
Dried fruit (raisins, prunes, apricots, etc.)	½ cup	¼ cup
100% fruit juice	1 cup	½ cup

SOURCE: USDA www.MyPyramid.gov

Sip vegetable soups and stews. Minestrone, split pea, tomato, black bean, lentil, hot and sour, gazpacho, pasta fagioli, chili, mushroom, vichyssoise, and butternut squash are just a few of the soup choices. When possible, make sure that cream-based soups are made with low-fat or nonfat ingredients to reduce calories. About one to one and a half cups of soup provide about one serving of vegetables.

Eat one-dish wonders. Salads, stir-fry, casseroles, spaghetti, lasagna, moussaka, and pizza are just a few that can come loaded with vegetables. There's a lot of variation here, but figure that one portion provides about a serving of vegetables—maybe more if you have a large entrée-size salad.

Soothe your sweet tooth with fruit. Doesn't matter if it's fresh, frozen, canned, or dried. One piece of fruit equals about a cup. So does a four-ounce container of applesauce, since it's more concentrated. A small box of raisins or other dried fruit (one-quarter cup) provides the equivalent of one-half cup of fruit or four ounces of fruit juice. Choose fruit—or vegetable—desserts whenever possible. A slice of pumpkin pie provides about one serving of vegetables. Lower the calories and fat by skipping the crust.

Washington, D.C.: I've recently rediscovered a great food—frozen grapes. I froze a bunch last week to snack on for dessert, and have found that if I am craving chocolate or ice cream, eating a couple of frozen grapes satisfies that craving.

Sally Squires: Great idea, D.C. Let me add frozen peaches—or any other slightly thawed frozen fruit—as another option. Top with two tablespoons of whipped cream (just 25 calories—be sure to measure) and a few slivered nuts for a great healthy dessert.

Drink your fruits and veggies. Fresh-squeezed juice has more pulp and fiber than commercial brands of juice. Plus, there's no added sugar. With an electric juicer you can make a glass in seconds. Limited time? Then look for unsweetened cranberry, blueberry, and other juices to make your own "juice cocktail." Warning: They're tart, but these unsweetened juices mix well with sweeter juices, such as orange or apple, or with sparkling water and a dash of lime. Tomato and V8 juice are other smart choices that clock in at just 35 calories per six ounces. (If you're worried about salt, choose the lower-sodium varieties.)

Slice and dice. It will add variety. So top your morning cereal with half a banana and some fresh berries. Grate apples on your oatmeal. Toss some mango slices or chopped pineapple or mandarin oranges in your salad. Throw some chopped tomatoes, mandarin oranges, onions, or water chestnuts into your tuna salad. Stir-fry with broccoli, cabbage, mushrooms, water chestnuts, and onions. The only limit is your imagination.

Roast a rainbow. Baking isn't just for your favorite roast beef. Roasted vegetables are a wonderful way to meet the daily requirements. Wash and cut vegetables—cubes of sweet potatoes, zucchini, tomatoes, whole mushrooms, slices of onions, garlic, sliced or whole sweet peppers. Place them in a nonstick roasting pan. Season with herbs, salt, and pepper to taste. Spray with olive oil or drizzle one or two tablespoons—depending on your calorie goals—and toss. Then bake at 350° until they are golden.

For a delicious dessert, grill peaches—yes, peaches!—sliced in half and placed on a grill that is sprayed with oil. Or try grilled grapes or other fruit. No grill? Pop them under the broiler or wrap in foil—bananas, pears, and apples are particularly good this way. Season with cinnamon and bake until they are caramelized. Yum.

Learning to savor food in this fashion is what helps Lean Plate Club members of all ages and sizes and from all geographic locations gradually instill healthier eating habits. As a member from North Carolina describes: "I graduated from college a year ago and decided to make the commitment to drop the 20 pounds that I gained during four years of cafeteria eating. I didn't want to start a diet and instead found a lot of information from the National Institutes of Health (www.nih.gov) and American Cancer Society (www.acs.org) about nutrition and weight loss. I am on a 1,400- to 1,500-calorie-a-day plan and have added in more consistent exercise with a pedometer.

DELICIOUS . . . AND MOST NUTRITIOUS

Fruits	Vegetables
Rich in vitamin A	
Apricots	Carrots
Cantaloupe	Collard greens
Mango	Pumpkin
	Spinach
	Sweet potatoes
	Turnip greens
Rich in vitamin C	
Cantaloupe	Broccoli
Citrus fruit and juice	Cabbage
Kiwi	Peppers
Strawberries	Potatoes
	Romaine lettuce
	Spinach
	Tomatoes
	Turnip Greens
Packed with folate	
Oranges and orange juice	Dried beans and peas
	Mustard greens
	Spinach
Packed with potassium	
Bananas	Greens, including spinach
Dried fruit	White or sweet potatoes
Orange juice	Winter (orange) squash
Plantains	

SOURCE: 2005 U.S. Dietary Guidelines

"In the beginning I had to count calories for everything (with help from online resources), but now I am really good at estimating. I have lost ten pounds so far in 12 weeks. I keep a weekly food/exercise diary. I really enjoy the Lean Plate Club and look forward to the tips from fellow participants. It helps keep me motivated to know others are out there."

PUT IT INTO PRACTICE
WHAT COUNTS AS 1 CUP OF VEGETABLES?

1 cup of raw or cooked vegetables or vegetable juice, or 2 cups of raw leafy greens can be considered equal to 1 cup from the vegetable group. Use this to find specific amounts that count as 1 cup of vegetables (in some cases equivalents for ½ cup are also shown) toward your recommended intake.

	Amount that counts as 1 cup	Amount that counts as ½ cup
Dark green vegetables		
Broccoli	1 cup chopped or florets	
	3 spears 5" long raw or cooked	
Greens (collards, mustard greens, turnip greens, kale, spinach)	1 cup cooked	
	2 cups raw	1 cup raw

(*continued*)

	Amount that counts as 1 cup	Amount that counts as ½ cup
Raw leafy greens (spinach, romaine, watercress, dark green leafy lettuce, endive, escarole)	2 cups raw	1 cup raw

Orange vegetables

	Amount that counts as 1 cup	Amount that counts as ½ cup
Carrots	1 cup strips, slices, or chopped, raw or cooked 2 medium 1 cup baby carrots (about 12)	1 medium about 6 baby carrots
Pumpkin	1 cup mashed, cooked	
Sweet potato	1 large baked (2¼" or more diameter) 1 cup sliced or mashed, cooked	
Winter squash (acorn, butternut, Hubbard)	1 cup cubed, cooked	½ acorn squash, baked = ¾ cup

	Amount that counts as 1 cup	**Amount that counts as ½ cup**
Dry beans and peas		
Dry beans and peas (black, garbanzo, kidney, pinto, or soybeans; black-eyed peas, split peas)	1 cup whole or mashed, cooked	
Tofu	1 cup ½" cubes (about 8 ounces)	1 piece 2½" × 2¾" × 1" (about 4 ounces)
Starchy vegetables		
Corn, yellow or white	1 cup	
	1 large ear (8"–9" long)	1 small ear (about 6" long)
Green peas	1 cup	
White potatoes	1 cup diced, mashed 1 medium boiled or baked potato (2½" to 3" diameter) French fried: 20 medium to long strips (2½" to 4" long)	
Other vegetables		
Beans, green or wax	1 cup cooked	
Bean sprouts	1 cup cooked	

(continued)

	Amount that counts as 1 cup	Amount that counts as ½ cup
Cabbage, green	1 cup, chopped or shredded, raw or cooked	
Cauliflower	1 cup pieces or florets, raw or cooked	
Celery	1 cup, diced or sliced, raw or cooked	
	2 large stalks (11"–12" long)	1 large stalk (11"–12" long)
Cucumber	1 cup raw, sliced or chopped	
Lettuce	2 cups raw, shredded or chopped	1 cup raw, shredded or chopped
Mushrooms	1 cup raw or cooked	
Onions	1 cup chopped, raw or cooked	
Peppers, green or red	1 cup chopped, raw or cooked	
	1 large (3" diameter, 3¾" long)	1 small
Tomatoes	1 large raw whole (3") 1 cup chopped or sliced, raw, canned, or cooked	1 small raw whole (2¼") 1 medium canned
Tomato or mixed vegetable juice	1 cup	½ cup
Zucchini or summer squash	1 cup cooked, sliced or diced	

SOURCE: USDA www.MyPyramid.gov

BUY SMART

Nothing takes the wind out of your efforts—or a bite out of your wallet—like stocking the fridge with fresh fruits and vegetables only to discover that they're wilted or growing fuzz by the time you eat them.

- **Fruits most likely to stay fresh in the fridge:** Apples, clementines, pears, oranges, grapes, lemons, limes, grapefruit, and tangerines.

- **Fresh vegetables with longest shelf life:** Cabbage; carrots; celery; cucumbers; iceberg lettuce (yes, it has nutritive value, although not as much as some other choices); romaine lettuce; root vegetables including potatoes, rutabagas, sweet potatoes; pumpkin; various types of squash.

- **Best buys:** Any fruits or vegetables in season plus canned or frozen vegetables, especially grocery stores' generic brands. Where possible, look for products without added sodium or sugar to keep calories lower. If that's not possible, rinse canned products several times to help reduce sodium.

Stretch your food dollars. Lean Plate Club members often save money—and expand their nutritional horizons—by shopping at food co-ops or farmers' markets, or by joining a Community Supported Agriculture program. To find CSA options near you, log on to www.nal.usda.gov/afsic/csa/csastate.htm.

Got a healthy, great-tasting recipe that you'd like to share? Send it to the Lean Plate Club Web chat at www.leanplateclub.com, where prizes are awarded every Tuesday to a handful of participants.

Recipes. Find a sampling of healthy recipes to help you boost consumption of fruits and vegetables in Chapter 15. The National Cancer Institute's 5 to 9 a Day program features a free online database of recipes to help you increase your intake of fruit and vegetables. You can search these recipes by ingredient, meal, preparation time, and number of servings of fruits and vegetables per person at www.5aday.gov/recipes/index.html. Or check out the free recipes rich in fruits and vegetables at the Produce for Better Health Foundation, a group sponsored by growers, grocery stores, and other industry groups interested in promoting greater consumption of fruits and vegetables: www.5aday.com/html/recipes/onthemenu.php.

Davidson, N.C.: One of the best things that I have learned in this process is to spread my calories throughout the day. Healthy snacks are a must for me. I also cook in quantity and then freeze in individual portions, so there is always something nutritious to pop in the microwave. I eat a lot of vegetarian meals, and here is a casserole I came up with recently.

VEGGIE ENCHILADA CASSEROLE

1 can black beans
1 can corn
½ can diced tomatoes with green chilies
½ bag frozen spinach (microwave and drain excess water)
1 cup low-fat Monterey Jack or Cheddar
1 can enchilada sauce
garlic powder
cumin
chili powder
cayenne pepper (if desired)

cilantro (fresh or dried)
cooking spray
9 small corn tortillas broken in pieces

1. Preheat the oven to 400°.
2. Combine the beans, corn, tomatoes, spinach, ½ cup cheese, and ½ can enchilada sauce in a bowl. Add spices to taste.
3. Spray a 9" × 13" baking dish with cooking spray.
4. Spread ½ of the remaining enchilada sauce in the baking dish. Top with ⅓ of the tortilla pieces. Cover with half of the veggie mixture. Add another ⅓ of the tortilla pieces. Layer with remaining veggie mixture. Top with the last of the tortillas, remaining enchilada sauce, and the remaining ½ cup of cheese.
5. Bake for 30 minutes, or until brown and bubbly.

Makes 6 servings of approximately 275 calories, perhaps more depending on the brands you use (I use tortillas that are 45 calories each).

ALL SIZES FIT

Over these next eight weeks, you'll discover how to identify real—versus perceived—hurdles to physical activity and how to add more physical activity whether you're currently a dedicated couch potato or a committed gym rat. Truth is, except for those training for the next Olympics, almost everyone needs to boost their daily activity.

Dear Sally: Thank you very much for your preaching about healthy lifestyle habits. On Saturday, I told my two girls, ages four and five, to get on their bikes, and I put my son in his stroller and off we went. It was so beautiful outside. I was so engrossed in its beauty that I walked for about an hour without feeling tired. My kids had such a nice time. We did it again the next day. We're going to do it again this weekend.

1. **Record the exercise that you get this week.** Use the form on page 143. Pay attention here: Don't alter your usual level of physical activity in any way. Behavioral research shows that if you begin two new habits together, when you slip—and believe me, we all slip up at some time—you're more likely to stop both new habits because they were started at the same time. So it's best to add just one new habit this week: Focus on eating more fruits and vegetables. Hold steady on whatever physical activity you're doing—or not doing—and keep to the calorie level that you've determined meets your needs.

2. **Pick up a pedometer.** It's an easy way to track how many steps you get daily. These tiny devices cost about $10 to $35, far less than a gym membership or even a weekly exercise class. They clip on to your belt or waistband. A pedometer will provide another measure of your daily activity and will serve as a handy reminder to move more. Here's what else you need to know about pedometers:

Wear it properly. Holding the pedometer in your hand won't do. Ideal placement is at the waist. Waistband too thick for the pedometer? Wear it on your underwear. Just make sure the pedometer is secure and horizontal. If your waistband is loose, your steps are likely to be underestimated. To avoid losing your pedometer, buy a model that offers a safety clip, or add your own.

Exercise Essentials

Begin to gather these items in the next week or two.

- Comfortable, well-fitting athletic shoes.
- Exercise clothes (T-shirt, shorts, tights, yoga pants—whatever fits you easily, breathes well, and feels good).
- Free weights or resistance bands. (Canned goods and milk or juice bottles with handles can also be used.)
- For women: supportive workout bra. Title 9 Sports (www.title 9sports.com) has a wide variety of large sizes and styles.
- Bathing suit (optional).

Check the accuracy of your pedometer. Some fancier models allow you to plug in your stride to the pedometer. You can change it for walking or jogging (which generally involves a longer stride). Whether yours allows you to do this or not, perform this simple test. Zero the pedometer. Place it on your body where you intend to wear it. Take 100 steps. If the pedometer reads between 90 and 110 steps, it's working properly. If it doesn't, move it to another part of your body and test again.

Other placement options are just beneath your navel, at your waist in the middle of your back, or (for women) in the middle of your bra. If the pedometer still doesn't measure accurately in any of those places, then you likely need a new pedometer.

No magic numbers. You've probably heard about taking 10,000 steps a day for weight loss. Don't worry about the numbers this week, other than to see how many steps you get in your usual routine. This is the time when you are establishing a baseline—the number of steps that you normally take right now. You'll have plenty of time in the coming weeks and months to boost your activity levels.

Pedometer accuracy varies widely. In a test of 13 pedometers published in a peer-reviewed scientific journal, University of Tennessee researchers found that the Kenz Lifecorder, Yamax Digi-Walker SW-200 and SW-701, New Lifestyles NL-2000, and Sportline 330 performed most accurately. University of Colorado researchers found that pedometers are most accurate at speeds of three miles per hour or more.

Pedometer Resources
- America On the Move, www.americaonthemove.org
- Accusplit, www.accusplit.com
- Digi-Walker, www.digiwalker.com
- Sportline, www.sportline.com

GOALS

Use the form provided on the next page to track your daily and weekly goals. Photocopy it and carry it with you for easy access. You'll find an updated form at the end of each week in the Lean Plate Club Program.

REWARD

Be sure to reward yourself when you achieve your goals this week. Make a contract now with yourself. When you complete your goals, give yourself a reward that you decide upon now. Write it here: _____. It could be a leisurely bubble bath by candlelight, an extra hour of sleep, a new CD you've wanted, or renting a workout tape at the local video store.

WEEK 1 GOALS

Monday   **Tuesday**   **Wednesday**   **Thursday**   **Friday**   **Saturday**   **Sunday**

Record calories. Stay at the daily calorie level for your goals:_____

☐   ☐   ☐   ☐   ☐   ☐   ☐

Add fruits and vegetables.

Fruit: _____ cups*/daily for your calorie level

☐   ☐   ☐   ☐   ☐   ☐   ☐

Vegetables: _____ cups*/daily for your calorie level

☐   ☐   ☐   ☐   ☐   ☐   ☐

*1-cup equivalents: 1 piece of fruit; 8 ounces of juice; $\frac{1}{2}$ cup dried fruit, 1 cup cooked or raw vegetables; 2 cups raw, leafy greens (lettuce, spinach, arugula); 1 small potato

Get a pedometer. Record how many steps you log daily.

_____   _____   _____   _____   _____   _____   _____

Track your physical activity but don't change anything yet.

Example: Monday

Walked the dog–10 minutes

Took stairs twice

Walked to errand–10 minutes

Shot hoops with kids–10 minutes

Total: 30 + minutes

Reward _____ **Earned** ☐

Seven

WEEK 2: FIBER UP!

Middle age is when you choose your cereal for the fiber, not the toy.

—*Anonymous*

If the mere mention of fiber makes you think only of eating bran, then you're in for a pleasant surprise. Fiber is found in a host of great-tasting foods, from crusty whole-grain baguettes to steamy bowls of oatmeal. Even those fruits and vegetables that you've indulged in this past week are often rich in fiber. So you're already ahead of the curve. And since fiber helps you feel full, you're likely to be satisfied with fewer calories, according to a number of research studies.

How much fiber you need daily depends on your age and your gender, but if you're like most adults, you fall short. Both men and women get only half the fiber they need, according to a large national survey of food intake by the U.S. Department of Agriculture.

Men aged 19 to 50 years need 38 grams of fiber daily. Those 51 and older need 30 grams of fiber per day. Women aged 19 to 50 years require 25 grams of fiber daily, while those 51 and older need 21 grams per day.

TO BOOST FIBER

Breakfast like a high-fiber champion. Make the right choice on your morning cereal and you could be halfway to your daily fiber goal. Cereals high in fiber include General Mills' Fiber One, Kellogg's 100 Percent Raisin Bran, Post's Shredded Wheat 'n Bran, and Post's 100% Bran Cereal. Can't stomach high-fiber cereals? Mix with regular cereal or fruit to help make the taste more palatable and gradually decrease the amount of lower-fiber cereal over time. That helps to ease into a higher-fiber cereal. And don't forget oatmeal. About one cup of cooked oatmeal will give you about four grams of fiber—two of those grams are good for your gastrointestinal tract; two help reduce blood cholesterol levels. Plus, there's new evidence to suggest that eating a breakfast of oatmeal with milk may help make you sharper than eating a bowl of sweetened ready-to-eat cereal.

JUST ½ CUP PACKS . . .

	Fiber (grams)
Cereal, 100% bran	10
Kidney beans, lentils, or split peas	8
Black, lima, or pinto beans	7
Chickpeas, navy, or white beans	6
Quinoa (whole grain)	5
Mixed vegetables	4
Raspberries or blackberries	4
Soybeans (edamame)	4
Bulgur wheat	4
Brown rice	2
Wild rice	1½

Switch to high-fiber grain varieties of bread, crackers, pasta, and rice. They have double or more the fiber found in the more highly processed white bread, pasta, and rice. Rye, pumpernickel, and other whole-grain breads are good choices, with about 3 grams per slice. Wild rice and brown rice also have about 3 to 4 grams of fiber per cup. Whole wheat pasta packs about 6 grams of fiber per cup. Always read the nutrition facts label, since it's the only way to know fiber content for sure. Case in point: Stone ground or multigrain does not necessarily mean whole wheat.

High-Fiber Brownies

Ingredients: Any commercial, regular-size brownie mix and one 15-ounce can black beans. Put undrained beans in food processor. Blend until smooth. Mix with the brownie mix. Bake as directed on the package. Cool and serve:

100 calories per brownie, 0 grams fat, 2 grams fiber.

Eat potatoes and fruits with the skin. This adds about a gram of fiber per serving.

Practice smart snacking. Choose popcorn (1 gram of fiber/cup) and other whole grains, as well as fruits and vegetables. Get 2 grams of fiber from a small banana, 3 grams from a medium apple with the skin or from ½ cup of cooked broccoli. A cup of berries provides 6 to 8 grams of fiber. A half cup of roasted soybeans has about 4 grams of fiber. One stalk of celery has about 1 gram of fiber. It all adds up.

Reach for beans. With up to 17 grams per cup, beans are fiber standouts. Two good options: baked beans (6½ grams per ½ cup), a bean burrito (about 6 to 8 grams of fiber) with a corn tortilla (for an extra gram of fiber), or bean soup. Plus, beans are rich in protein, complex carbohydrates—which won't make blood sugar soar—and iron.

WHAT ABOUT FIBER SUPPLEMENTS?

Day after day, commercials and ads promote fiber products—Citrucel, Fibercon, Benefiber, and Metamucil—that promise to deliver the benefits of healthy fiber without even having to chew.

EAT JUST ONE AND YOU'LL GET

	Fiber (grams)
Artichoke	6
Mestemacher bread, slice	6
Sweet potato, medium (with skin)	5
Guava, medium	5
Apple (with skin)	4
Pear, small	4
Pita bread, whole wheat, medium	3
Whole wheat English muffin	4
Potato, medium (with skin)	4
Banana, medium	3
Orange	3

SOURCES: 2005 Dietary Guidelines Advisory Committee Report and Nutrition Facts Labels

---

Do they beat the healthful benefits of eating high-fiber foods? Not likely, because none of them are meant to be used daily but rather for short periods of time, about a week.

Fiber supplements also provide just a single source fiber instead of the mix delivered naturally in food. Plus, most of the fiber supplements don't pack the vitamins, minerals, and healthful phytonutrients that high-fiber food provides.

Some people—for example, those on early phases of very low-carb diets, such as Atkins or South Beach, or the elderly—may have eating habits that make it difficult to get enough fiber in their diets. In that case, experts say that fiber supplements may be helpful for short periods of time to promote regularity.

SNACKS

	Fiber (grams/ounce)
Snyder's of Hanover Soy Teins	5
GO LEAN Roll Bars	5
Larabar	5
Popcorn	4
Terra Chips	3
Dried apricots (¼ cup)	3
Wasa Fibre Rye	3
Wasa Hearty Rye crackers	2
m&m's with peanuts	2

For most people, it's easy to meet the daily goal with food if you know a few high-fiber secrets:

- Start the day with high-fiber cereal topped with fruit.

- Order your sandwich at lunch on whole wheat bread.

- Have a bean salad, vegetarian chili, bean soup, or a bean burrito (up to 17 grams per cup) for dinner to meet or even exceed the daily recommendations.

- Snack on fruits and veggies and you've got it made. (Check out the numbers in the table on pages 149–151.)

FIND YOUR FAVORITE HIGH-FIBER FOODS

The leading source of fiber in today's diet is bread, according to national food surveys. While bread is a fine food, you can find lots of other opportunities to add variety, flavor, and high fiber to your daily fare. Here's a list of the foods that pack the most fiber. Photocopy it. Choose your favorites and use it to help guide you in adding more fiber to your daily food repertoire.

PUT IT INTO PRACTICE
HOW TO GET ENOUGH FIBER DAILY? EASY!

Breakfast:

High-fiber cereal	8–14 grams/cup
Berries	8 grams/cup

Snack:

Apple, large (with skin)	5

Lunch:

Whole wheat bread in sandwich	3 grams/slice

Snack:

Bean dip with whole wheat crackers	4–6 grams

Dinner:

Bean burrito	7 grams

Total: 35–43 grams

FIBER FACTS

	Fiber	Calories
100% bran ready-to-eat cereal (½ cup)	10	78
Kidney beans, canned (½ cup)	8	109
Split peas, cooked (½ cup)	8	116
Lentils, cooked (½ cup)	8	115
Black beans, cooked (½ cup)	8	114
Pinto beans, cooked (½ cup)	7	120
Lima beans, cooked (½ cup)	7	108
Artichoke globe, cooked	7	60
White beans, canned (½ cup)	6	154
Chickpeas, cooked (½ cup)	6	135
Great Northern beans, cooked (½ cup)	6	105
Navy beans, cooked (½ cup)	6	129
Cowpeas, cooked (½ cup)	6	100
Soybeans, mature, cooked (½ cup)	5	149
Bran ready-to-eat cereals, various, 1 ounce	3–5	91–105
Rye wafers, plain, 2	5	74
Guava, 1 medium	5	46
Sweet potato, baked, with skin, 1 medium	5	131
Asian pear, raw, 1 small	4	51
Green peas, cooked (½ cup)	4	67
Whole wheat English muffin, 1	4	134
Pear, 1 small	4	81
Bulgur, cooked (½ cup)	4	76
Mixed vegetables, cooked (½ cup)	4	59
Raspberries, fresh (½ cup)	4	32
Sweet potato, boiled, no skin, 1 medium	4	119
Blackberries, fresh (½ cup)	4	31
Potato, baked, with skin, 1 medium	4	240
Soybeans, green, cooked (½ cup)	4	127
Stewed prunes (½ cup)	4	133

	Fiber	Calories
Figs, dried (¼ cup)	4	93
Dates (¼ cup)	4	126
Oat bran, raw (¼ cup)	4	58
Pumpkin, canned (½ cup)	4	42
Spinach, frozen, cooked (½ cup)	4	30
Almonds, 1 ounce	3	164
Apple with skin, fresh, 1 medium	3	72
Brussels sprouts, cooked (½ cup)	3	33
Whole wheat spaghetti, cooked (½ cup)	3	87
Banana, 1 medium	3	105
Orange, 1 medium	3	62
Oat bran muffin, 1 small	3	178
Pearled barley, cooked (½ cup)	3	97
Sauerkraut, canned (½ cup)	3	23
Tomato paste (¼ cup)	3	54
Winter squash, cooked (½ cup)	3	38
Broccoli, cooked (½ cup)	3	26
Shredded wheat ready-to-eat cereals, various, 1 ounce	2–3	78–95
Parsnips, cooked (½ cup)	3	55
Turnip greens, cooked (½ cup)	3	24
Collards, cooked (½ cup)	3	25
Okra, frozen, cooked (½ cup)	3	26
Peas, cooked (½ cup)	3	42

PUT IT INTO PRACTICE
EASY STEPS TO INCREASE ACTIVITY

1. Get off the elevator one or two floors early and walk the rest of the way.
2. Pick up lunch a block or two away from the office.
3. Deliver messages in person instead of by e-mail.
4. Make multiple trips to carry small loads of groceries or laundry rather than one large load.
5. Use a drinking fountain or restroom on another floor.
6. Set a timer every hour during the workday. When it goes off, take a two- to five-minute walk around the office and reset for another hour. Repeat throughout the day.
7. Walk the sidelines of your kids' sports games and practice instead of sitting. Or do laps around the field or gym, or climb the bleachers.
8. Keep a pair of comfortable walking shoes in your car and/or desk to take a quick stroll.
9. Recruit a workout buddy to jog, walk, go to the gym, or take an exercise class.
10. Take the stairs whenever possible.
11. Walk—don't stand—on escalators or moving walkways.
12. Change the television channels manually rather than using the remote.
13. Pace while brushing your teeth or drying your hair.
14. Vacuum and dust your house as many times as possible during the week, even if you have a cleaning person or service.
15. Use your feet—not the car—to walk or bike to as many errands as possible.
16. Mow your lawn with a walking, rather than a riding, mower. If your yard is large, use the mower for only part of the yard.
17. Put on your favorite CD or get out your iPod and dance while you're waiting for dinner to cook.

18. Shoot hoops with your kids.
19. Use manual appliances whenever possible: can openers, whisks, etc.
20. Get a "jogging" stroller to walk your kids to the park and playground, rather than drive.

ALL SIZES FIT

This week's physical activity goal is to add just a two-minute walk per day on top of whatever else you're doing right now. And no, this alone won't get you or anyone else in shape to run a marathon or compete in the next Olympics. But numerous studies show that small, incremental additions to daily activity develop into bigger long-term habits. View this as just the first step toward adding physical activity above your baseline last week. On your pedometer, aim for 1,000 more steps per day than last week.

As a Lean Plate Club member from Maryland, who once experienced shortness of breath from doing household chores and now regularly bikes 60 miles in a day, notes: "Exercise is cumulative. Stick with it. Walking those two blocks will turn to four and eight and more and pretty soon your entire cardiovascular system will have expanded and improved to the point where you'll be able to exercise even longer. Your fitness level will grow steadily until, one day, you'll be able to look back to how you feel today and see how far you've come."

WEEK 2 GOALS

Monday	Tuesday	Wednesday	Thursday	Friday	Saturday	Sunday

Record calories. Stay at the daily calorie level for your goals:_____

☐   ☐   ☐   ☐   ☐   ☐   ☐

Fruit and vegetables

Fruit: _____ cups*/daily for your calorie level

☐   ☐   ☐   ☐   ☐   ☐   ☐

Vegetables: _____ cups*/daily for your calorie level

☐   ☐   ☐   ☐   ☐   ☐   ☐

*1-cup equivalents: 1 piece of fruit; 8 ounces of juice; $\frac{1}{2}$ cup dried fruit; 1 cup cooked or raw vegetables; 2 cups raw, leafy greens (lettuce, spinach, arugula); 1 small potato

Add fiber (25 grams a day for women and 38 grams a day for men 50 and younger; 21 grams per day for women and 30 grams per day for men 51 and older).

Your daily goal: _____

☐   ☐   ☐   ☐   ☐   ☐   ☐

Add 2-minute walk/day.

☐   ☐   ☐   ☐   ☐   ☐   ☐

How many steps did you average each day last week? _____

+ 1,000 steps/daily

_____

Daily steps goal this week: _____

Reward _____ **Earned** ☐

Eight

WEEK 3: SWAP THE BAD FOR THE GOOD

Jack Sprat could eat no fat,
His wife could eat no lean;
And so betwixt the two of them,
They licked the platter clean.
>   *—17th-century English nursery rhyme*

After years of being demonized and misunderstood, fat has come back into favor. Not only is "fat-free" often not much of a calorie saver (as you'll find in the table on page 156), but healthy fats are good for you. So good that the 2005 Dietary Guidelines, the American Heart Association, and other groups advise consuming *more* healthy fat.

Here's where it can get tricky: Since healthy fat contains the same 9 calories per gram as all other fats, it needs to be eaten both sparingly and wisely. **The secret: Swap the bad for the good wherever possible and keep a careful eye on the bottom line.**

SECRET: FAT-FREE—NOT ALWAYS THE SMART CHOICE

	Calories		Calories
Reduced-fat peanut butter, 2 T	187	Regular peanut butter, 2 T	191
Fat-free fig cookies, 2 (30 g)	102	Regular fig cookies, 2 (30 g)	111
Nonfat vanilla frozen yogurt (< 1% fat), ½ cup	100	Regular whole-milk vanilla frozen yogurt (3–4% fat), ½ cup	104
Fat-free caramel topping, 2 T	103	Caramel topping, homemade with butter, 2 T	103
Low-fat blueberry muffin, small (2½")	131	Regular blueberry muffin, small (2½")	138
Low-fat cereal bar, 1 (1.3 oz)	130	Regular cereal bar, 1 (1.3 oz)	140

SOURCES: Nutrient Data System for Research, version v4.02/30, Nutrition Coordinating Center, University of Minnesota; National Heart, Lung, and Blood Institute; National Institutes of Health

Reach for healthy fat first. By all means, have a few slices of avocado on your sandwich. Top your salad with slivered almonds. Stir-fry your asparagus in a tablespoon or two of olive oil. Sprinkle a little wheat germ on your breakfast cereal. Grind some flaxseed into your pancakes. Snack on a couple of olives or a handful of nuts. Drizzle a little olive oil and vinegar on your salad. These oils are rich in healthy monounsaturated and polyunsaturated fats and contain very little unhealthy, artery-clogging saturated fat or trans-fatty acids.

Secret: To cut saturated fat, skip the solids:

Beef fat (tallow, suet)

Butter

Chicken fat

Pork fat (lard)

Stick margarine

Shortening

SOURCE: USDA www.MyPyramid.gov

Get oily. Replace butter and other saturated fat with healthy oils. Olive, canola, corn, cottonseed, soybean, and safflower oils are just a few smart choices. Check out specialty oils such as peanut, walnut, hazelnut, macadamia, and, if you really want to splurge, try truffle oil, which has a slightly musty flavor. Just remember to swap—not add—these oils for less healthy fat, while staying within your daily calorie goals. For most sedentary people, that means a total of about two tablespoons (six teaspoons) daily for salad dressings, sauces, cooking, and the margarine that you slather on your morning toast. If you're more active—30 minutes daily or higher—you may be able to add a little more healthy fat.

HOW MUCH IS MY DAILY ALLOWANCE FOR OILS?

You can get plenty of healthy oil in foods, especially

- nuts
- fish
- cooking oil
- salad dressings

How much you need depends on your age, gender, and level of physical activity.*

Women

19–30 years	6 teaspoons
31+	5 teaspoons

Men

19–30 years	7 teaspoons
31+	6 teaspoons

SOURCES: USDA www.MyPyramid.gov

*These amounts are appropriate if you get less than 30 minutes per day of moderate physical activity beyond your normal daily activities. If you're more physically active, you may be able to consume more while still staying within your calorie goals.

PUT IT INTO PRACTICE
HOW DO I COUNT THE OILS I EAT?

The table gives a quick guide to the amount of oils in some common foods.

	Amount	Amount of oil	Calories from oil	Total calories
Oils				
Vegetable (canola, corn, olive, peanut, safflower, soybean, sunflower)	1 tablespoon	3 teaspoons	120	120

	Amount	Amount of oil	Calories from oil	Total calories
Foods				
Almonds, dry roasted	1 ounce	3 teaspoons	130	170
Avocado	½ medium	3 teaspoons	130	160
Cashews, dry roasted	1 ounce	3 teaspoons	115	165
Hazelnuts	1 ounce	4 teaspoons	160	185
Italian dressing	2 tablespoons	2 teaspoons	75	85
Margarine*	1 tablespoon	2½ teaspoons	100	100
Mayonnaise	1 tablespoon	2½ teaspoons	100	100
Mayonnaise-type salad dressing	1 tablespoon	1 teaspoon	45	55
Mixed nuts, dry roasted	1 ounce	3 teaspoons	130	170
Olives, ripe, canned	4 large	½ teaspoon	15	20
Peanut butter	2 tablespoons	4 teaspoons	140	190
Peanuts, dry roasted	1 ounce	3 teaspoons	120	165
Sunflower seeds	1 ounce	3 teaspoons	120	165
Thousand Island dressing	2 tablespoons	2.5 teaspoons	100	120

*Soft, trans fat–free margarine

Look at your bottom line. No need to get so obsessive that you count fat by the gram, but it's still smart to track roughly how much you consume. Keep measuring spoons handy. Use them to portion out the oil you use to sauté your spinach, make your salad dressing, and measure the peanut butter for your PB&J sandwich.

Somewhere: Hi, Sally. I've noticed some products say they have no trans fats, in which case they usually list "trans fats 0 grams" in the nutritional information. But I don't understand how to tell if products have it or not. I thought maybe there were trans fats in partially hydrogenated oils, but my "Oatmeal and Fruit" bars say "Trans Fats 0 grams" and also list "partially hydrogenated soybean oil" in the ingredients. What's the deal, do you know?

Sally Squires: On January 1, 2006, the FDA began requiring that food manufacturers list trans fats on nutrition facts labels. Partially hydrogenated oils *do* contain trans fats. But foods with less than 0.5 gram per serving can be labeled as having zero trans fats.

You should also know that some products listing partially hydrogenated fat contain only trace amounts of trans fats. That's because trans fats form during deodorization of vegetable oils, a process that is nearly impossible to avoid.

Best bet: Read nutrition labels carefully for grams of fat. Reach for foods with the lowest amounts of trans and saturated fats. One additional clue: The higher that partially hydrogenated oils are listed on ingredients labels, the greater the potential for trans fats.

Choose margarine and margarine-like spreads wisely. They can be sources of unhealthy trans fats. Smart choices include Promise, Take Control, Smart Balance, and Benecol. Take Control, Benecol, and Smart Balance Omega Plus Buttery Spread also contain plant stanols and sterols that when used regularly can help lower blood cholesterol as much as some cholesterol-lowering drugs. Moderation is still key, however, since healthy margarines contain as many calories—about 70 to 80 per tablespoon—as regular margarine. Unlike some stick margarines, tub varieties generally contain no trans fats. To save calories, choose light versions, which run about 50 calories per tablespoon.

Nibble nuts. They have vitamin E and plenty of healthy fat, but eat them judiciously, since at nearly 200 calories per ounce—equal to about a handful—they can pack a lot of hidden calories. Slice, sliver, and dice to get the great flavor and the health benefits of nuts with fewer calories.

Measure!

Free-pouring olive oil without measuring can add lots of extra calories.

1 tablespoon	120 calories
½ cup	1,000
1 cup	2,000

SOURCE: USDA

Easy on the bread and oil. It's become standard practice at many restaurants to deliver a basket of warm bread and some olive oil for dipping to diners. Delicious? Yes. Caloric? You bet. While waiting for the meal, it's easy to consume 400, 500, even 600 calories from the oil alone. So have a slice of bread—not half the basket—then use your teaspoon to measure and drizzle a small amount of olive oil on the bread. Or order shrimp cocktail, smoked oysters, or trout—other great appetizers that are also sources of healthy omega-3 fats.

Polyunsaturated Fats

What the experts say: Replace saturated and trans fats with polyunsaturated fats.

Good choices: Canola, soybean, safflower, sunflower, corn, and peanut oils.

Limit saturated fat to less than 10 percent of total daily calories, (200 calories—about 22 grams of fat—on 2,000 calories/day), since there's no evidence of safety for higher levels.

Think outside the bottle and tub. A Canadian Lean Plate Club member who has lost more than 100 pounds in the past two years describes how she has altered her use of healthy oils: "I have found that a lot of recipes that have butter oil or fat might not need it. For frying, try a spray, or just use water or water and broth. You only need a little to steam something. I have a bread machine cookbook that replaces butter with applesauce, and the bread came out great. I also have recipes where I used fat-free sour cream instead of margarine, and the cake came out moist. And I've used cocoa instead of chocolate, and it was a delicious chocolate cake. I do eat about two teaspoons of healthy oil daily, such as olive, safflower, or canola oil. I have also cooked with light margarine or just used a couple teaspoons of it with good results."

Small changes added up to big rewards for her—and can for you, too.

Go for variety. It's just as important with healthy fat as it is with other foods. A few examples: Sesame oil contains phytosterols, which can help lower blood cholesterol. Soybean oil has carotenoids, which are converted in the body to vitamin A. Rice bran oil has the antioxidant oryzanol.

Secret Way to Burn More Calories

"More Is Burned as Energy. Not Stored As Fat." That's what Enova oil, made by ADM KAO, one of the newest healthy oils, promises. But does it really do that?

Enova is a reformulated mixture of soybean and canola oils that is rich in digyclerides, a kind of fat that is not easily sent to fat cells by the body. So it's transported to the liver instead, where Enova is burned for energy. Could that translate to more lost pounds if Enova is used in place of other oils?

Maybe. But the evidence is still emerging.

One published study found a trivial two-pound weight loss in a group of overweight people who averaged 200 pounds and used the oil for three months. If you decide to use Enova, here's what you need to know:

- **Proceed cautiously.** Since Enova contains the well-known canola and soybean oils, it is being sold under an FDA provision known as GRAS, or "generally recognized as safe." It has not yet undergone extensive testing in the United States, although it has been used in Japan since 1999.
- **Don't expect to save calories.** Like other liquid oils, Enova has 120 calories per tablespoon, so it's no caloric bargain. Enova is meant to replace other oils, not add to them.
- **Great for baking, not for dipping.** Enova has no flavor, so you probably won't relish dipping bread in it the way you might virgin olive oil. But it seems to earn high marks in salad dressings, sautéed food, and baked goods.

Find omega balance. A century ago, most fat came from free-range animals, which had higher levels of healthy omega-3 fatty acids than the mass-produced beef, poultry, and pork commonly eaten today. Soybean oil—now one of the leading fats in processed foods—accounted for just 0.02 pound per year of fat. That all changed in the 1960s when soybean oil saturated the U.S. food chain. Today, it's a major ingredient of crackers, bread, salad dressing, baked goods, and other processed food, accounting for 20 percent of the total calories consumed in the United States, according to the U.S. Department of Agriculture. Per capita consumption is about 25 pounds per year—more than 1,000 times higher than a century ago. Some experts think this shift is a bad idea, since omega-6 fatty acids compete against omega 3s for use by the body. Until scientists sort it out, boost omega-3 consumption when possible, which can also help cut heart disease risk.

Fat Secrets

Add: Almonds, avocados, sunflower seeds and oil, canola oil, hazelnuts, Brazil nuts, pine nuts, peanuts, peanut butter and oil, flaxseed oil, olives and olive oil, healthy margarine (without trans fats)

Limit: Butter, heavy cream, sour cream, whole-milk yogurt, whole-milk products including whole-fat cheese, egg yolks, margarine with trans fats (in commercially prepared baked goods and some frozen foods)

Avoid: Partially hydrogenated and hydrogenated oils

Give oil longer shelf life: Exposure to air causes oxidation. Once opened, store in a cool, dark place. Keep walnut, flaxseed, and other specialty oils in the refrigerator.

Where to get monounsaturated fat:

- Canola oil
- Olives and olive oil
- Safflower oil
- Sunflower seeds and oil

Many low-calorie plant foods also have omega-3 fatty acids, including flaxseed, cantaloupe, arugula, chicory, collard greens, kale, mustard greens, purslane, Swiss chard, wild greens, and mungo beans (a lentil-like bean popular in Indian cuisine.) But the omega 3s found in fish and seafood are easiest for the body to use.

Fats

Omega 6 (Linoleic Acid)
What the experts say: Replace saturated and trans fats with polyunsaturated, where possible.

Adequate daily intake: men, 17 grams/day, about the amount found in 3 pats of margarine or 4 Hershey's Kisses or 1 slice of American Deli Deluxe Cheese; women, 12 grams/day or the amount found in 3 Hershey's Kisses or 3 FritoLay Rold Gold Pretzels or 2 pats of margarine

Where to get it: soybean, corn, and safflower oils

SOURCE: National Academy of Sciences; Penny Kris-Etherton, Ph.D., Pennsylvania State University

---

Auburn, Ala: I am a vegetarian. Is eating tofu and nuts good enough, or should I try to use a supplement to get omega 3s? Also, is it important to eat walnuts as opposed to other nuts?

Sally Squires: No fish? You can help boost omega 3s by eating

- Wild rice
- Kidney beans
- Melon
- Spinach
- Cauliflower
- Broccoli
- Boston lettuce
- Gouda cheese
- Cherries
- Grape leaves
- Mungo beans

All have good ratios of omega-3 to omega-6 fatty acids—although they still fall short compared with fish. Flaxseed oil is another good choice, as is olive oil, which is not rich in omega 3s but doesn't come loaded with omega 6s.

SOURCE: Keep It Managed (KIM), National Institutes of Health

Make smart substitutions. Snacking on a small amount of nuts and dried fruit instead of a candy bar can be a good trade-off, but switching from a low-fat turkey sandwich to a tuna salad sandwich slathered with mayo may not be, even though both the tuna and the mayo contain healthy types of fat. The tuna salad sandwich starts at 700 calories. With extra mayo, it can climb to 800. Compare that to the turkey sandwich, which clocks in at about 370 calories.

WHAT'S BETTER: BUTTER OR MARGARINE?

	Saturated Fat (grams)	Trans Fats (grams)	Calories (per tablespoon)
Butter	7	0	100
Tub margarine	1½	0	80

SOURCE: U.S. Food and Drug Administration

ALL SIZES FIT

Boost activity five minutes per day over what you were doing during Week 1. And yes, if this sounds tiny, it is. The point is to slowly get into the habit of daily activity, even if it's just a small amount. If you want to do more, go for it. Just be sure that you make the daily goal. Consistency is the only way really to gain a new habit. Even if you already work out regularly at the gym, or take daily jogs or walks, odds are you're probably pretty sedentary the rest of the day. So yes, this added five minutes is for you, too.

- Skip delivery takeout and walk to pick up lunch at a restaurant at least five blocks from your office. And walk back.

WALKING! Hi, Sally—My sister is participating in a study that's looking at a link between getting 10,000 steps a day and weight loss. She wears a pedometer and writes down how many steps she logs daily. She does pretty well but usually has to walk on the treadmill to get in enough steps each day. Except when we went sightseeing and ended up walking 20,000 steps in one day!

WALK ¼ MILE IN 5 MINUTES

Weight (pounds)	Calories burned
130	16
145	18
164	20
190	24
220	27

SOURCE: Calories Per Hour (www.caloriesperhour.com)

- Take the long way into your building from the parking lot.

- Get off the bus or subway a stop early and walk the rest of the distance. Or walk to a farther stop before getting on public transportation.

- Ride an exercise bike or walk a treadmill, stair machine, or elliptical trainer for five minutes while watching a television program.

- Put on two or three of your favorite fast tunes and dance to them nonstop.

- Set a timer and see how much you can vacuum in five minutes.

- Rake the yard or sweep the front steps or sidewalk for five minutes.

Cambridge, Mass.: I recently brought my cholesterol down by 40 points by going on a "good fat" diet, which let me eat lots of things that I love so I didn't feel deprived. Like: salad with avocados and cold-pressed extra virgin oil (and balsamic vinegar), peanut butter, nonfat whole wheat breads, Take Control spread, chocolate soy milk, dried pineapples, trail mix, sk n milk lattes, etc.

WEEK 3 GOALS

Monday	Tuesday	Wednesday	Thursday	Friday	Saturday	Sunday

Record calories. Stay at the daily calorie level for your goals:_____

☐   ☐   ☐   ☐   ☐   ☐   ☐

Fruit and vegetables

Fruit: _____ cups*/daily for your calorie level

☐   ☐   ☐   ☐   ☐   ☐   ☐

Vegetables: _____ cups*/daily for your calorie level

☐   ☐   ☐   ☐   ☐   ☐   ☐

*1-cup equivalents: 1 piece of fruit; 8 ounces of juice; $\frac{1}{2}$ cup dried fruit; 1 cup cooked or raw vegetables; 2 cups raw, leafy greens (lettuce, spinach, arugula); 1 small potato

Fiber (25 grams a day for women and 38 grams a day for men 50 and younger; 21 grams per day for women and 30 grams per day for men 51 and older)

Your daily goal: _____

☐   ☐   ☐   ☐   ☐   ☐   ☐

Replace saturated and trans fats with healthy fat (2 servings† per day).

☐   ☐   ☐   ☐   ☐   ☐   ☐

†A serving could be 2–3 ounces of fish or seafood (175–225 calories); $\frac{1}{3}$ cup nuts (200 calories); 2 tablespoons of peanut butter (190 calories); $\frac{1}{2}$ cup tofu (100 calories); $\frac{1}{4}$ avocado (90 calories); 1 tablespoon of salad dressing made with canola, olive, safflower, or other healthy oil (80–120 calories); 1 tablespoon of Take Control or Benecol.

Add 5-minute walk/day.

☐   ☐   ☐   ☐   ☐   ☐   ☐

How many steps did you average each day last week?   _____

+ 1,000 steps/daily

_____

Daily steps goal this week: _____

Reward _____ **Earned** ☐

Nine

WEEK 4: PROTEIN POWER

If you pay even slight attention to nutrition news and trends, you have heard about protein bars, protein shakes, protein powders, and yes, even the promises of high-protein diets to help pounds "melt away." Although these claims exaggerate what protein can do, it's true that the body does use a little more energy to burn protein than either carbohydrates or fat. Before you get too excited, the rev in metabolism is small. More interesting is the emerging evidence that suggests increasing protein intake can give you a slight edge in feeling full, certainly a benefit when you're trying to reach a healthier weight.

University of Washington researchers led by physician Scott Weigle put a group of slightly overweight men and women on a low-fat, higher-protein regimen with plenty of healthy carbohydrates. The researchers found that when they boosted protein to about twice as high as what Americans usually eat—that's equal to an extra serving or two of lean chicken breasts—participants spontaneously decreased what they ate by nearly 500 calories per day. Even more interesting: Participants had no hunger pangs but rather reported feeling full and satisfied. And anticipating your question, they lost weight, too. (Find some of the recipes used in the study in Chapter 15.)

Just as there are many types of fats and carbohydrates, so, too, is there a wide range of protein, so you'll have plenty of choices.

In fact, there's more variety with protein than with either carbohydrates or fat.

POTENT PROTEIN

Fish, lean meat, poultry, and other animal products are the most complete protein that gives you all nine indispensable and essential amino acids. No need, however, to be a carnivore to get the protein required: Eggs, milk, cheese, yogurt, and plenty of plant-based foods, from black beans to the soybean-based tempeh and tofu, all contain protein. Even carbohydrates—from apples to bread to zucchini—contain small amounts of protein and underscore the nutritional value of eating a wide variety of foods.

Here's how to get the most punch from your protein.

Protein

What the experts say: Get 10 to 35 percent of daily calories as protein.

	Daily amount (ounces)
Men	
19–30 years	6½
31–50	6
51+	5½
Women	
19–30 years	5½
31+	5

SOURCES: National Academy of Sciences Dietary Reference Intakes, Macronutrients; USDA

A little goes a long way. Just 3 ounces of lean meat or poultry contain about 25 grams of protein, about half the daily recommendation. You can get 20 grams of protein from 3 ounces of fish or in 1 cup of soybeans. Dairy food is another great source of protein. A glass of skim milk provides 8 grams. An egg or 1 ounce of cheese contains about 6 grams of protein.

Have your daily bread. Sure, bread is filled with carbohydrates, but dense, whole-grain breads provide as much as 5 grams of protein per slice—or about 10 percent of the daily recommendation. Other surprising protein sources include whole-grain cereals and vegetables, with about 2 grams of protein per ½-cup serving. Some high-protein cereals contain double or triple that amount or more.

Protein Supplements?

Sure, you can shell out money to buy protein powder, bars, and drinks, but they don't necessarily mirror the protein found naturally in food and may come with extra saturated fat and added minerals that may be difficult to absorb. Get your protein and other vitamins and minerals from food.

Have an extra helping of beans. They're cheap, versatile, and filled with protein. One cup of black beans rivals the protein in a three-ounce chicken breast or a quarter-pound burger and has about three times the protein of a large egg.

"REDUCED GAS" BEANS

1. Place dry beans in hot water (10 cups per pound of beans).
2. Heat water to boiling and boil beans for 2 to 3 minutes.
3. Remove from heat, cover, and set aside for 1 to 4 hours. (The longer the soak time, the more sugars dissolve, making digestion easier.) Discard water before cooking beans.

SOURCE: California Dry Bean Advisory Board

Enjoy eggs. Because of cholesterol fears, eggs fell out of favor, but they're staging a comeback. Eggs are a good, inexpensive source of protein, with all the essential amino acids, iron, and lutein—which may help protect vision. Australia's National Heart Foundation—the equivalent of our American Heart Association— has recently given eggs a "check mark," signifying that they are a heart-healthy food for people without elevated blood cholesterol levels or heart disease.

Worried about cholesterol? Use egg substitutes or egg whites. One white contains about four grams of protein—about 10 percent of what a woman needs daily and about 9 percent of a man's intake—with zero fat and no cholesterol. So chop up boiled egg whites and add to salads. Or make "deviled" eggs filled with hummus, guacamole, or low-fat dip while avoiding added cholesterol.

Falls Church, Va.: I make a one-egg omelet in the microwave with salsa made fresh with tomatoes, garlic, red onions, cilantro, and jalapeño. It smells wonderful, and it is one more way to have an extra serving of vegetables, as well as protein. Add cheese—low-fat or nonfat—if you like.

Choose nonfat or low-fat dairy products. One cup of nonfat fruit yogurt has 11 grams of protein. A cup of skim milk has 8 grams of protein and zero fat. Other good choices are low-fat buttermilk and nonfat and low-fat yogurt and cheese. String cheese has about 80 calories per ounce, 8 grams of protein, and 5 grams of fat. New varieties of nonfat and low-fat cheese expand your options, especially for snacks and grilled cheese sandwiches, and clock in at about 35 to 40 calories per slice or wedge. Look for nonfat feta cheese, which has a hearty flavor. Or, for a protein boost, add nonfat dried milk to puddings and casseroles. Use nonfat milk to make creamy soups such as tomato, or oatmeal and other hot cereals.

Chicago, Ill.: I've lost 45 pounds in the last eight months and we eat out all the time. Almost every day for breakfast, I order an egg-white omelet with feta cheese and vegetables (either spinach or mixed broccoli, tomato, onion, mushroom). I get it cooked in Pam and have half a plain English muffin. OJ and coffee, too.

Add soy. Tofu, soy nuts, high-protein soy cereals, and soy-based meat substitutes add protein without adding a lot of fat. One slice of tofu contains 6 grams of protein. A quarter cup of dry-roasted soybeans packs 17 grams of protein, about a third of the daily requirement. A soy burger has 12 grams of protein and just 4 grams (or less) of fat. Add powdered soy protein, such as Genusoy, to orange or other juice for increased protein.

Fish for nutrition. Low in calories—unless it's deep-fat fried—rich in flavor, and filled with healthy omega-3 fatty acids, seafood is a good source of protein that also helps lower blood pressure, improves artery health, reduces triglycerides (blood fats linked to increased heart disease risk), and cuts the odds of developing a common, fatal irregular heartbeat. It also decreases formation of blood clots, which are linked to heart attacks and strokes. The American Heart Association recommends eating at least two servings of fish per week. Three ounces of salmon provide 17 grams of protein with just 5 grams of healthy fat.

High-Protein Snacks

- Cup of bean soup with nonfat cheese on top
- Handful of soy nuts
- Wedge of Laughing Cow cheese on a slice of cucumber, tomato, or an endive leaf
- Half a peanut butter sandwich on whole-grain bread
- Smoothie made with nonfat yogurt and fruit
- Glass of chocolate soy milk
- Any bean dip with veggies
- String cheese
- Smoked fish with nonfat cream cheese on whole-grain cracker
- Turkey, salmon, or beef jerky
- Barbecued tofu
- Energy bar
- Slices of fruit (apple/banana) with almond or peanut butter
- Hard-boiled egg (for lower cholesterol, fill yolk with salsa)
- Half cup high-protein cereal with skim milk and slivered nuts
- Pudding made with skim milk
- Kefir
- Low-fat buttermilk
- Celery stalk filled with low-fat cheese or peanut butter
- Shrimp cocktail

BEST PROTEIN SOURCES

Animal Protein

1 ounce of protein = 1 ounce lean meat, poultry without the skin, fish; ¼ cup cooked dry beans; 1 egg; 1 tablespoon peanut butter; ½ ounce nuts or seeds.

Eggs

Whole
Whites
Yolks
Egg substitutes

Fish and Shellfish

Anchovies
Catfish
Clams
Cod
Crab
Crayfish
Flounder
Haddock
Halibut
Herring
Lobster
Mackerel
Mussels
Octopus
Oysters

Pollack
Porgy
Salmon
Sardines
Scallops
Sea bass
Shrimp
Snapper
Squid (calamari)
Swordfish
Trout
Tuna

Meat

Beef
Arm pot roast
Bottom round roast
Brisket, flat half
Chuck shoulder roast
Eye of round
Flank steak
Ground (91 percent lean or higher)
Rib steak
Ribeye steak
Round tip roast
Shank crosscuts
T-bone steak
Tenderloin steak
Top loin (strip) steak
Top round steak
Top sirloin steak
Tri-tip roast

Game Meats
Bison
Rabbit
Venison

Lamb
Arm
Leg
Loin

Organ Meats
Giblets
Liver

Pork
Canadian bacon
Ham (fresh and cured center cut)
Loin chops
Tenderloin

PUT IT INTO PRACTICE
DRY BEANS AND PEAS

2 ounces protein = ½ cup dried beans

1 cup bean soup

1 soy burger

4 tablespoons hummus

2 ounces cooked tempeh

1 falafel patty

½ cup baked beans

½ cup refried beans

½ cup tofu

Poultry *(without skin)*
Chicken
Chicken sausage, lean
Cornish hens
Ground chicken
Turkey (except self-basting)

Plant Protein

Bean burgers and other meat substitutes
Black beans
Black-eyed peas
Chickpeas (garbanzo beans)
Falafel
Kidney beans
Lentils
Lima beans (mature)
Navy beans
Pinto beans
Seitan (wheat gluten)
Soybeans
Soy hot dogs
Soy sausage
Split peas
Tempeh (cultured soybeans with chewy texture)
Texturized vegetable protein
Tofu (bean curd made from soybeans)
Veggie burgers
White beans

Nuts and Seeds
Almonds
Cashews

Hazelnuts
Mixed nuts
Peanut butter
Peanuts
Pecans
Pistachios
Pumpkin seeds
Sesame seeds
Sunflower seeds
Walnuts

Since protein comes in many forms from beans and eggs to porterhouse steak, nuts, milk, and salmon, it can sometimes be confusing to know what counts as an ounce of protein. One ounce of protein equals

- 1 ounce of meat, poultry, or fish

- ¼ cup of cooked dry beans

- 1 egg

- 1 tablespoon of peanut butter

- ½ ounce of seeds or nuts

- 1 cup of nonfat milk

- 1 ounce of cheese

But since steak and burgers, shrimp cocktail, omelets, and chili rarely come in simple portion sizes, here's a guide to show you how much protein you'll likely get in some common foods.

WHAT COUNTS AS AN OUNCE OF PROTEIN?

	1-ounce equivalents	What you're more likely to find
Meats	1 ounce cooked lean beef	1 small steak (eye of round, fillet) = 3.5–4 ounces; 1 small lean hamburger = 2–3 ounces
Poultry	1 ounce cooked chicken or turkey (without skin)	½ small chicken breast = 3 ounces; ½ Cornish hen = 4 ounces
Fish	1 ounce cooked fish or shellfish	1 can tuna drained = 3–4 ounces; 1 salmon steak = 4–6 ounces; 1 small trout = 3 ounces; 7 large shrimp = 1 ounce
Eggs	1 egg 2 egg whites ¼ cup egg substitute	1 omelet = 2–3 eggs; scrambled eggs = 2 eggs
Nuts and Seeds	½ ounce nuts (12 almonds or 24 pistachios or 7 walnut halves)	1 handful nuts = ½–1 ounce

(continued)

	1-ounce equivalents	What you're more likely to find
Nuts and Seeds	½ ounce seeds (such as hulled and roasted pumpkin, sunflower, or squash seeds)	1 handful seeds = ½–1 ounce
	1 tablespoon of peanut, almond, or other nut butter	peanut butter sandwich = 2–4 tablespoons
Dry Beans and Peas	¼ cup cooked dry beans	1 cup bean soup = 2 ounces
	¼ cup tofu	stir-fry tofu at a restaurant = ¼–½ cup; 1 soy burger = 2 ounces
	1 ounce tempeh	vegetarian salad
	¼ cup roasted soybeans	about a handful
Dairy*	1 cup milk	small carton of milk
	1 ounce cheese	1-inch cube of cheese

SOURCE: USDA www.Pyramid.gov

*Recommendations are to consume at least 3 servings of milk or dairy products in addition to protein requirements.

ALL SIZES FIT

Increase physical activity to ten minutes per day above your baseline—that works out to a total of one hour per week above what you were doing when you started a few weeks ago. Sure, you can do more if you want. The point is that by slowly building in more physical activity to your daily life, you're building a habit—just like brushing your teeth.

And no, ten minutes a day certainly won't make you an Olympic athletic, but there's a growing body of scientific evidence that suggests these small bouts of activity pay off. Big-time.

At the University of Virginia, exercise physiologist Glenn A. Gaesser, Ph.D., has developed the Spark—ten-minute workouts that have been proved to boost cardiovascular fitness, strengthen muscles, and whittle waistlines. Similar research at the University of Pittsburgh, Maastricht University in the Netherlands, and elsewhere points to the value of brief bouts of physical activity. Even just doing this small amount of extra activity puts you well above the national curve. According to the 2005 Dietary Guidelines Report, 38 percent of adults—about four in every ten—engage in no leisure-time physical activity.

Ormond Beach, Fla.: To fit in more physical activity each day, I never stay sitting during the commercial breaks on TV. And that doesn't mean that I head for the fridge. During a break I can shake out throw rugs, put dishes into the dishwasher, quick-wipe the bathroom sink, etc. You get the idea.

What you decide to do is your call. Just make it a physical activity that you enjoy and can do consistently.

WEEK 4 GOALS

| Monday | Tuesday | Wednesday | Thursday | Friday | Saturday | Sunday |

Record calories. Stay at the daily calorie level for your goals:_____

☐   ☐   ☐   ☐   ☐   ☐   ☐

Fruit and vegetables

Fruit: _____ cups*/daily for your calorie level

☐   ☐   ☐   ☐   ☐   ☐   ☐

Vegetables: _____ cups*/daily for your calorie level

☐   ☐   ☐   ☐   ☐   ☐   ☐

*1-cup equivalents: 1 piece of fruit; 8 ounces of juice; ½ cup dried fruit; 1 cup cooked or raw vegetables; 2 cups raw, leafy greens (lettuce, spinach, arugula); 1 small potato

Fiber (25 grams a day for women and 38 grams a day for men 50 and younger; 21 grams per day for women and 30 grams per day for men 51 and older)

Your daily goal: _____

☐   ☐   ☐   ☐   ☐   ☐   ☐

Healthy fat (2 servings† per day)

☐ ☐   ☐ ☐   ☐ ☐   ☐ ☐   ☐ ☐   ☐ ☐   ☐ ☐

†A serving could be 2–3 ounces of fish or seafood (175–225 calories); ⅓ cup nuts (200 calories); 2 tablespoons of peanut butter (190 calories); ½ cup tofu (100 calories); ¼ avocado (90 calories); 1 tablespoon of salad dressing made with canola, olive, safflower, or other healthy oil (80–120 calories); 1 tablespoon of Take Control of Benecol.

Boost protein (20–35 percent of your daily calories: 100–175 grams on 2,000 calories per day).

☐   ☐   ☐   ☐   ☐   ☐   ☐

Add 10-minute walk/day.

☐   ☐   ☐   ☐   ☐   ☐   ☐

How many steps did you average each day last week? _____

+ 1,000 steps/daily

_____

Daily steps goal this week: _____

Reward _____ **Earned** ☐

Suitland, Md.: I have a sedentary job. To increase my physical activity, while at work I take a stair break every few hours. I go to a restroom on a lower floor and take the stairs back to my office. Sometimes I take the elevator down to the lobby and take the stairs back—I work on the 14th floor. I also park on the upper level of the garage and take the stairs to get to my car, which is at the far end of the garage! I've noticed that my breathing is getting better.

Ten

WEEK 5: CLEAN UP YOUR CARBS

Man does not live by bread alone.
　　　　　　　　　　　—*Moses*

What the late diet doctor Robert Atkins showed the world is that we often overeat carbohydrates or, more precisely, processed carbs. Those are the kind with white flour, little fiber, and often a lot of sugar.

Cake, cookies, bread, crackers, pasta, cereal, rice—processed carbohydrates are among the tastiest and most popular foods. There's nothing wrong with them in moderation. The challenge is to find that middle ground. Whole grains can help. They're the healthy carbs, the ones with fiber and more complex sugars that won't send your blood sugar soaring.

Two simple questions can help guide you:

- Is a food naturally sweet, or does it contain added sugar?

- Does it contain highly processed flour or at least some whole grains?

Take a crusty French baguette, a bowl of unsweetened whole-grain cereal, and a sugary meringue. They're all carbohydrate-rich food, but they deliver very different nutritional punches.

Carbohydrates

What the experts say: *Recommended dietary allowance* = 130 grams of carbohydrates for adults and children.

Food translation: 2 large apples + 3 slices of whole wheat bread = 130 grams of carbs.

Aim for: Keep carbohydrates at about 45–65 percent of calories daily, including 3 servings of whole-grain foods.
  On 2,000 calories per day that = 225–325 grams

SOURCES: 2005 Dietary Guidelines Committee Report; National Academy of Sciences Advisory Dietary Reference Intakes, Energy, Carbohydrate, Fiber, Fat, Fatty Acids, Cholesterol, Protein, and Amino Acids

---

The cereal comes loaded with complex carbohydrates that take longer to break down into simple sugars and so are less likely to raise levels of blood sugar or overtax insulin production. It also packs fiber and a little protein. Compare that to the baguette, with its highly processed white flour, and the meringue, which is loaded with refined sugar. Both are easy to digest and have little if no fiber to slow their progress through the digestive system. They're both quickly broken down into one of the simplest sugars—glucose—which prompts a spike in production of insulin. Though the bread's enriched flour provides some iron and a little folic acid, neither bread nor meringue can match the vitamins and minerals found in the cereal.

This doesn't mean that you should never eat French baguettes or meringues or even white bread. (More on that below.) Here's how to reach for more healthy carbs.

Grab some fruits and vegetables. They are prime sources of healthy carbs. To help keep their nutritional quotient as high as possible, choose whole fruit (canned, fresh, or frozen) over more highly processed versions with added sugar and fat. Ditto for vegetables. Baked potatoes are better than French fries or potato chips. A fresh orange is a better choice than orange juice. Baked apples or unsweetened applesauce is wiser than apple pie, which is of course a great treat for special occasions.

Add three whole-grain servings daily. The 2005 Dietary Guidelines Committee said this amount enables you to cover the nutritional bases. The U.S. Dietary Guidelines Scientific Advisory Committee underscored the nutritional importance of eating whole grains. Among the benefits: B vitamins, magnesium, iron, zinc, vitamin E, and antioxidants.

Look for golden stamps to help guide you. Developed by the Whole Grains Council, a consortium of chefs, industry scientists, and the Oldways Preservation Trust, a Boston-based nonprofit organization, the stamps will point you to "good" products that provide half a serving of whole grains; "excellent," those foods that give you a full serving of whole grains; and "100 percent," products that contain a full serving of whole grains and have no refined grains. To find out which foods have earned the stamps, log on to www.wholegrainscouncil.org.

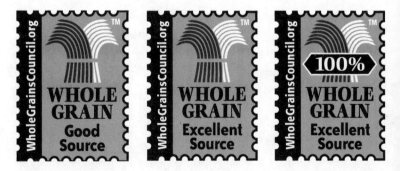

Used by permission of the Whole Grains Council and the Oldways Preservation Trust

Reach for the familiar. Healthy carbs don't have to be exotic. They can be as familiar as unsweetened shredded wheat, Wheaties, Total, and original Cheerios. There are whole-grain pretzels. Such favorites as Wheat Thins now come in a whole wheat variety. Triscuits have always been whole-grain and now contain no unhealthy trans fats.

Eat pasta al dente. When pasta is slightly undercooked, the starches in it are broken down less. Though it sounds like nutritional heresy, it's okay to go with white pasta. If you love whole wheat, that's a good choice, too, but there's no need to force yourself to eat it. Pasta is a dehydrated food that doesn't make blood sugar levels rise very high. In fact, it boosts them much less than white bread does. Whole wheat pasta simply has wheat bran added in such small amounts that it doesn't have any measurably different effect on blood sugar levels than white pasta.

Have another serving of dairy products. They contain lactose, a carbohydrate that is not sweet and doesn't raise blood sugar as much as other sugars. Of course, in keeping with the goal of swapping saturated fat for healthy fats, you'll also want to choose nonfat or low-fat dairy products.

Whole Wheat and White?

It sounds like a nutritional oxymoron, but a growing number of bakers are using winter white wheat to make whole wheat white bread. It has the same nutritional punch as standard whole wheat but with a milder flavor and a color that rivals traditional white bread. Brands to look for: Sara Lee's Soft & Smooth Made with Whole Grain White Bread, Sara Lee and Wonder Bread Whole Grain White Bread, and Wonder White Bread Fans 100% Whole Grain.

Or make your own: King Arthur Flour's white whole wheat product is sold in grocery and specialty stores and on the Web at www.kingarthurflour.com.

Eat your daily bread. Adding whole grains to your diet is as simple as picking out whole wheat bread at the grocery store. Just make sure it's really whole wheat. Bread made from "wheat flour" doesn't make the cut as a whole grain. "Whole wheat flour," "whole rye," "whole oats," or other "whole" grains need to be listed first or second on the ingredients list. A few smart choices are Arnold 100 Percent Whole Wheat, Mestemacher Rye Bread, and Pepperidge Farm 100 Percent Whole Wheat Bread.

Washington, D.C.: I'd tried using bulgur wheat a few times but always abandoned it because it tasted too bland. I recently discovered that if I use slightly less water to soak the bulgur and then add a can of fire-roasted diced tomatoes (with juice), the bulgur soaks up the tomato juice and is much more tasty.

I use one cup of bulgur soaked in ¾ cup of water, then add a 15-ounce can of fire-roasted tomatoes and their juice, the juice of one lemon, some chopped parsley, and some chopped peppers or celery. I add some chopped walnuts and nonfat yogurt for protein. It makes a complete lunch.

Start your day with oatmeal. Whether it's instant, steel cut, quick, or just plain rolled, this staple is 100 percent whole-grain. Oatmeal has 147 calories and 4 grams of fiber per cup. About half that fiber helps protect the heart and the rest helps keep things regular. Plus Tufts University researchers have found that children who had a bowl of oatmeal made with milk for breakfast performed better on tests in school than those who ate a bowl of Cap 'n Crunch cereal with milk. Particularly improved was spatial memory—important for art and helpful with some math and science. Similar studies point to memory improvement for adults who eat whole-grain, low–glycemic index foods such as oatmeal for breakfast.

Corvallis, Ore.: I switched to whole grains last year, and I've really enjoyed the taste and texture of these healthier products.

Right now, I'm having fun with what I call my Festival of Brown Rices. In addition to regular long-grain brown rice, the dry bulk food sections of local stores have brown basmati, brown jasmine, and brown short-grain rice. Exploring products that are new to me really adds variety and enjoyment to my largely vegetable-based diet.

And on the vegetable side, I'm also celebrating my Festival of Winter Squash. Each week, I come home from the farmers' market with a different winter squash: festival, delicata, sweet dumpling, sugar loaf, butternut, spaghetti . . . and I haven't tackled the big boys (banana, Hubbard, and the range of pumpkins) yet. I haven't met a squash yet that didn't taste yummy mashed with a sprinkling of granulated garlic or Parmesan, or a spoonful of low-fat cottage cheese.

Go beyond brown rice. Barley, bulgur wheat, and buckwheat are whole grains. So is whole wheat couscous, quinoa, and amaranth. Whole-corn tortillas are a whole-grain product. If your family's palate needs a chance to adjust, start by mixing white rice with brown rice, etc., to ease into whole grains. Or make half-and-half sandwiches with one slice of whole wheat, one slice of white.

Snack well. Ryvita, Ak-Mak, Wasa, and Ry-Crisp are whole-grain crackers. Such popular crackers as Triscuits and Wheat Thins now come in whole-grain versions. Barbara's makes a whole-grain "saltine." Kashi has a whole line of whole-grain crackers. The list goes on and on. Graham crackers can be another option, provided that the first ingredient is graham flour, not enriched flour. Taco chips are made from whole grains but also often contain added fat and salt. Don't be fooled by "degerminated cornmeal," which is not a whole grain. Whole-wheat pita bread is another whole-grain option. Dip it into hummus for a good snack. Or use slices of red pepper, baby carrots, and celery as ways to eat bean dip or guacamole, a source of healthy fat. Trade your fruit juice for low-sodium vegetable juice. And when you're tempted to have a more processed sweet treat, make it a small one with a mix of sugar, healthy fat, and protein, such as M&M's with peanuts.

High-fiber, multigrain, and cracked wheat don't mean whole-grain. Example: 100 percent bran is a good source of fiber, but it's not a whole grain. Bran is just one part of the whole grain, which also includes the endosperm and the germ, the prime ingredient in wheat germ. Multigrain and cracked wheat suggest whole grain but often are not. Check the label to be sure.

Enjoy popcorn. This popular food is a whole grain. Just go easy on the salt and butter. That also goes for commercially prepared varieties, whether bought at the movie theater or put in the microwave. A lot of that may come loaded with salt, saturated fats, and trans fats.

New Albany, Ind.: Here's a whole-grain soup recipe that is easy, quick, and inexpensive. Great as a meal opener, side dish, or main supper with a great salad.

BULGUR SOUP

28 ounces canned crushed or pureed tomatoes
6 cups water or vegetable broth
1 small onion, finely chopped
1 cup bulgur
½ teaspoon oregano
herbs as desired, such as basil
salt and pepper to taste

Place all the ingredients in a large pot and cook 25 minutes over medium heat.

Sip your whole grains. Make your own whole-grain soup with the broth of your choice, some frozen vegetables or canned beans, and brown or wild rice. Or try the commercially prepared brands, including Frontier Soup's Iowa Open House Grain Pasta Potage, Montana High Plains Wheat Berry Chili, and Washington State Lentil Cracked Wheat (www.frontiersoups.com).

Mix it up. If you can't live without a sesame bagel, Rice Krispies, or white rice, simply add foods that will help mute the blood sugar rise from more processed fare. Eat Rice Krispies with skim milk, berries, and a few nuts. Spread low-fat cream cheese—not nonfat, which raises blood sugar more—on just half a bagel and add a slice of smoked salmon. Eat white rice with plenty of vegetables and a little lean meat, poultry, fish, or beans.

Rocky Hill, N.J.: I started with whole grains by doing a 60-40 mix of regular–whole grain (for example, white and brown rice). I then gradually increased the whole grain and decreased the regular. By the time I was at 100 percent brown rice, I was hooked.

ALL SIZES FIT

This week's activity goal is to maintain the minimum daily activity goal of ten minutes. Let me underscore again: This alone will not get you in peak physical shape. What you're doing, however, is gradually making physical activity a daily habit, just the way that brushing your teeth is part of your regular routine. In the coming weeks and months, you can gradually increase your workout time and try lots of different activities. Even now, if you either are more fit or find you want to do more than this minimum, that's fine. In fact, it's wonderful. Just be sure that you get in the ten minutes every day without fail, no matter what else you do.

The second physical activity goal is to begin weight training three times per week. Also known as strength or resistance training, lifting weights not only strengthens muscles but also is proved to build bone and even rev metabolism—a little. It's a valuable activity for toning and strengthening no matter what your age or fitness level.

What may be more important is what University of Connecticut exercise physiologist William Kraemer, Ph.D., editor in chief of the *Journal of Strength Training and Conditioning Research,* calls the "after-burn" of strength training. Just 15 minutes of weight training can burn 100 to 200 calories in the 24 hours after a workout. Since experts recommend weight lifting every other day—that respite enables affected muscles time to recover—regular workouts could allow you to burn an extra 300 to 600 calories a week.

Mix Up Your Workouts

Take a tip from the University of Connecticut Human Performance Lab, where workouts are designed to be light, medium, and heavy to build muscle more efficiently and avoid boredom.

Each workout takes 10 to 15 minutes. Lift weights every other day to give muscle time to recover and rebuild. Or if you want to lift daily, do upper body one day, lower body the next.

- *Light workout:* Use weights that you can lift 12 to 15 times (repetitions or reps, for short). Do 2 sets.
- *Heavy workout:* Use weights that you can lift only 3 to 5 times. Do 3 sets.
- *Medium workout:* Lift weights that are in between your light and heavy weights. So if you use 15-pound weights for heavy days and 5-pounds for light days, choose 8- to 10-pound weights for medium days. Do 3 sets of 8 to 10 reps.

SOURCE: William Kraemer, Ph.D., University of Connecticut Human Performance Laboratory

---

Near the end of this chapter, you'll find some simple weight-training activities to get you started. They range from abdominal crunches and chair stands to biceps curls. That's just the beginning. You'll find more weight-training sources on page 196.

In the meantime, keep these things in mind when beginning strength training:

Go slowly. You want to avoid injury and build a habit that you can sustain long term. This isn't a race. Figure that it takes about two months of regular conditioning to really get up to speed with weight lifting, particularly if you have been sedentary. So start with light free weights—about 3 to 8 pounds for women, about 5 to 10 pounds for men—and slowly build up.

Choose your venue. Sure, you can join a gym, but you can also do plenty of weight-resistance training at home or even at the office. Freestanding weights are inexpensive and can be bought individually or in sets. Don't want to invest in weights? Start by lifting canned goods. Or try resistance bands.

Use your own body weight. Jumps, push-ups, abdominal crunches, and pull-ups are other ways to do weight training. All help build muscle by working against your body weight. Everybody needs power, whether it's to stand up from a chair, unload groceries, work in the yard, climb the stairs, do the laundry, or just lift your bag to the overhead luggage compartment on an airplane. Power exercises, such as jumps, can also build bone, as British researchers learned when they had 75-year-old women jump in the air 50 times a day. People with knee, hip, or spinal problems should check with their doctors first, of course.

Lift the right amount of weight for you. Younger athletes tend to go too heavy; older athletes often go too light and may miss 65 to 75 percent of the possible benefits of weight training. Experts say that the upper limit for weights should be what you can comfortably lift three to five times in each of three sets. And

---

Additional Weight-Training Resources

- Collage Video, www.collagevideo.com. View free clips of exercise videos before you buy them. Among top-rated strength-training workouts are *The Firm*, Kathy Smith's *Lift Weight to Lose Weight 2*, and Tamilee Webb's *I Want That Body!*
- Magazines, including *Fit*, *Men's Health*, *Self*, *Shape*, *Prevention*, *Women's Health*, and *More*, frequently offer weight-training exercises in their pages and on their Web sites. Use them to help keep your workout fresh.
- Netflix, www.netflix.com. Rent weight-lifting DVDs, and have them delivered to your door via mail. Other types of workouts are available, too.
- Video Fitness, www.videofitness.com, offers reviews of a wide variety of fitness tapes/DVDs, plus viewer forums and more. Also, since the site only reviews, but doesn't sell, workouts, no need to worry about any conflict of interest.

---

ladies, don't worry about building too much muscle, because women lack enough of the male hormone testosterone required to do that.

Listen to your body. Good pain is when you're working hard and feel tired. Bad is any sharp physical pain. Stop immediately. Of course, it's always best to check with your physician before starting any exercise program and to take the PAR-Q test found on page 52. Before starting any weight-lifting program, be sure to ask your physician if you have any internal organic or musculoskeletal problems that prohibit your participation.

Carlisle, Pa.: I just wanted to let you know that I have now lost a total of 20 pounds following Lean Plate Club advice—15 to 30 minutes on the exercise bike most weekdays, and 15 minutes of moderate weight training/ab work for two to three evenings per week. I am scheduled for my first physical in several years and am looking forward to hearing good news about such things that I don't readily measure (cholesterol, blood pressure). I've had some ups and downs, but remembering your "one step today" advice and knowing that healthy habits beget more healthy habits has been a big help. Thanks, Sally and LPC!

Consistency is key. Results take work and dedication. Even health professionals can slip into bad habits and get out of shape. After studying and counseling athletes for years, the University of Connecticut's William Kraemer realized that he had let himself go. As he approached his fiftieth birthday, Kraemer put his own research into practice. He started weight training and other regular cardio exercise. He also got his eating habits back in order. The result: Kraemer trimmed 50 pounds, one for each of those birthday years he celebrated.

Princeton, N.J.: When on a low-carb diet, should I follow the "net carbs" or the "carbs" on the packaging? I'm completely confused.

Sally Squires: You're not alone. In fact, Atkins Nutritionals, Inc., which coined the term "net carbs," has now dropped the term. While there wasn't an official FDA definition for net carbs, Atkins and other food companies calculated a product's net carbs by subtracting grams of fiber and sugar alcohols from the total carbohydrate grams. The idea was to help higher-carbohydrate foods appear to have lower amounts of "net carbs." Don't worry about them.

WEIGHT TRAINING

Weight training takes practice to get the right form, which is why it's best to learn the activities and then gradually increase the weight lifted (or, if you're using resistance bands, to go to stronger bands).

This is one activity where it can be worth it to have a session with a physical trainer. Many gyms offer weight-training instruction as part of their regular membership practice. If you go this route, take notes. Ask for additional help if you're ever uncertain of a move or not sure how to use a weight machine. If you do use weight machines in a gym, it's common courtesy to wipe down the machine after you're finished for the next user.

The exercises included here are just a sampler of weight-training activities. Consider them appetizers to whet your appetite. They will help get you started, but they are not meant to sustain you.

Check your PAR-Q test results before beginning these or any other physical activities. Consult first with your doctor if you have any current or chronic health problems.

Other resources for weight training include:

- **American Academy of Orthopedic Surgeons,** "Beginning a Weight Training Program," at http://orthoinfo.aaos.org/fact/thr_report.cfm?Thread_ID=149&topcategory=Sports%20%2F%20Exercise.

- **American Council on Exercise.** This is the largest nonprofit fitness and certification provider in the world. Download dozens of exercises from agility and balance to resistance training from their free online fitness library at www.acefitness.org/getfit/freeexercise.aspx.

- **Centers for Disease Control and Prevention,** "Growing Stronger: Strength Training for Older Adults." This free, interactive Web-based program includes animation, three stages

of activities, and a booklet that can be downloaded. Go to
www.cdc.gov/nccdphp/dnpa/physical/growing_stronger/
exercises/more_exercises.htm.

- **National Institute on Aging** publishes "Exercise: A Guide" on
  www.niapublications.org/exercisebook/ExerciseGuideComplete
  .pdf. This free online program includes information on how
  to exercise safely, as well as activities to maintain endurance,
  strength, balance, and flexibility.

Warm Up

Before beginning any weight or resistance training, be sure to
warm up with at least five to ten minutes of brisk walking either
outdoors, indoors, on a treadmill, or in place. Using a stationary
bike, elliptical trainer, stair climber, or rowing machine are other
ways to warm muscles before doing weight training. These activities help to increase blood flow to the muscles to prepare them for
training. The following exercises were developed by the National
Institute on Aging.

Chair Stand

This helps strengthen your abdominal and thigh muscles, which are
known as core muscles. Do this exercise without using your hands as
you become stronger. Place a pillow on a chair, as shown. Sit toward
the front of the chair, with your knees bent and feet flat on floor.

Lean back on the pillow in a half-reclining position. Keep your
back and shoulders straight throughout the exercise. Raise your upper body forward until you are sitting upright, using your hands as
little as possible (or not at all, if you can). Your back should no
longer lean against the pillow.

Slowly stand up, using your hands as little as possible. Slowly
sit back down. Pause. Repeat 8 to 15 times. Rest, then do another

set of 8 to 15 repetitions. As you become stronger, you can start in the standing position with your arms held out in front of you. Bend as if to sit, stopping just about an inch above the chair seat. Then rise. Repeat 8 to 15 times. Rest. Repeat.

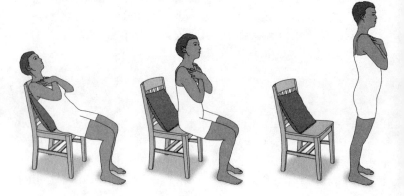

Arm Raise

Sit on an armless chair with your back supported by the back of the chair. Keep your feet flat on the floor. Hold hand weights straight down at your sides, with your palms facing inward.

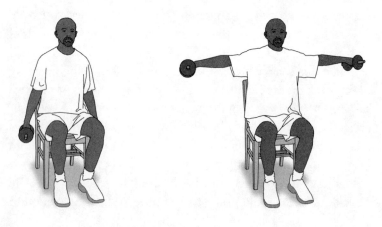

Raise both arms sideways to shoulder height. Hold for one second. Slowly lower your arms to your sides. Pause. Repeat 8 to 15 times. Rest, then do another set of 8 to 15 repetitions.

Abdominal Curl

Lie on your back on the floor with either both knees or one knee bent. Keep your feet flat on the floor. Pull in your stomach so that your back is flat on the floor.

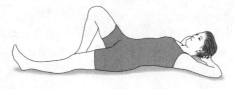

Place your hands behind your head, elbows pointing out. Slowly raise your shoulders and upper back off of the floor to the count of two. Pause. Slowly lower your shoulders back to the floor to the count of two. Repeat ten times for one set. Rest for one to two minutes. Then complete a second set.

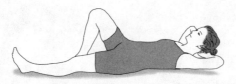

Tips: Don't hold your breath during this exercise. Exhale as you raise and inhale as you lower. Avoid pulling your head or neck with your hands and arms. Make the movement with your abdominal muscles. Keep your chin and eyes pointed toward the ceiling and your elbows pointed out—not up—throughout the exercise.

Side Leg Raise

This exercise helps strengthen the muscles at the sides of your hips and thighs. Stand straight, with your feet slightly apart. Hold on to a table or chair for balance. Slowly lift one leg 6 to 12 inches out to the side. Keep your back and both legs straight. Don't point your toes outward; keep them facing forward. Don't strain or arch your back. Keep your stomach muscles tight, trunk upright. Hold the position for one second. Slowly lower your leg. Pause. Repeat with the other leg. Alternate legs until you have done 8 to 15 repetitions with each leg. Rest, then do another set of 8 to 15 alternating repetitions. When you are ready, use ankle weights to increase intensity.

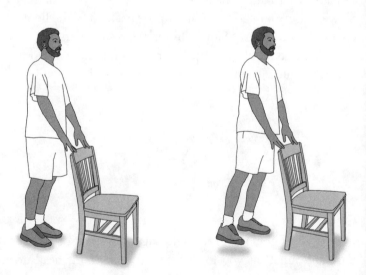

Biceps Curl

With a dumbbell in each hand, sit in an armless chair, with your feet shoulder-width apart, arms at your sides, and palms facing your thighs. (You can also stand if you prefer.)

Slowly lift the weights so that your forearms rotate and your palms face in toward your shoulders. Keep your upper arms and elbows close to your sides—as if you had a magazine tucked beneath each arm. Keep your wrists straight and the dumbbells parallel to the floor. Pause. Then slowly lower the dumbbells back toward your thighs, rotating your forearms so that your arms are again at your sides, with your palms facing your thighs. Repeat ten times for one set, with a count of two to raise the weights and a count of four to lower them. Rest for one to two minutes. Then complete a second set of ten repetitions.

Tip: Keep your elbows tight against your body and your wrists straight.

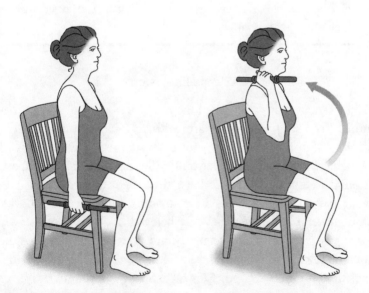

Mid-Atlantic state.: I concur with the slow and steady approach to gaining muscle. I am a 53-year-old woman. Last summer, I decided my upper-body strength needed a lot of help. At first I could not do a single "real" push-up (I did do the modified ones from my knees); it took me almost a month to be able to do one. At six months I could do 10 to 15. In another six months, I got up to 30 to 35 push-ups. So it took a long time, but I have eventually gotten a lot stronger. I do other exercises, but the progress has been most trackable with the push-ups.

The most remarkable thing I have found from getting stronger is how much better it makes me feel all day long. For a long time, I didn't think it was all that important. I really don't care if I can lift heavy stuff and I don't care a lot about how my arms look. But I was surprised how gaining abdominal and arm and chest and back strength improved my posture and just the way I feel—I sit and move more comfortably, I even think I feel taller! So I highly recommend doing some strength exercises for the way you will feel, never mind any weight-loss benefits (which are small) and looks (I do think I look better, too!).

Triceps Extension

This exercise helps strengthen the muscles in back of your upper arms. Keep supporting your arm with your hand throughout the exercise. Sit in a chair with your back supported by the back of the chair. Place your feet flat on the floor shoulder width apart. Hold a weight in one hand. Raise the weight toward the ceiling, your palm facing in. Support your arm lifting the weight with your other hand, placing it just below the elbow. Now slowly drop your arm with the weight toward your back. Then raise the weight toward the ceiling by straightening your arm. Hold the position for one second. Slowly bend your arm toward your shoulder again. Pause. Repeat the bending and straightening 8 to 15 times. Repeat 8 to 15 times with your other arm. Rest, then do another set of 8 to 15 alternating repetitions.

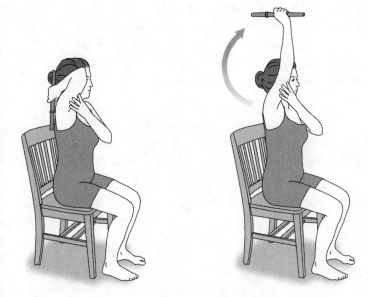

Wall Push-Up

Standard push-ups are a great way to strengthen your arms and core trunk muscles, but many sedentary people don't have the muscle strength to do them properly. Start to strengthen your muscles with wall push-ups, which will gradually strengthen

---

New Jersey: Down 16 pounds in the past five months and hope that when I weigh in tomorrow, I will hit my first goal—the loss of 10 percent of my weight. While I belong to Weight Watchers, much of my success comes from regular Lean Plate Club

(continued)

reading. The commonsense, real-food approach really is best and most satisfying.

So muscle building—good old-fashioned crunches done with a stability ball and push-ups—has shown amazing results. While I eat better, do aerobics, and see the weight falling steadily, until I started these, the results showed on the scale and not anywhere else. I don't yet have Madonna's arms or abs, but I see the difference, and it feels wonderful to boot!

---

your arms, shoulders, and chest. When you're ready, progress to modified push-ups on your knees and slowly work up to the full push-up.

Find a wall that is clear of any objects—wall hangings, windows, etc. Stand a little farther than arm's length from the wall. Face the wall. Lean forward and place your palms flat against the

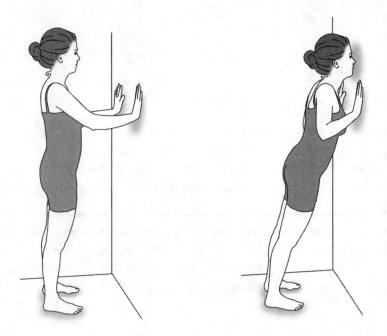

wall at about shoulder height and shoulder width apart. To a count of four, bend your elbows as you lower your upper body toward the wall in a slow, controlled motion. Keep your feet firmly planted on the floor. Pause. Then, to a count of two, slowly push yourself back until your arms are straight—but don't lock your elbows. Repeat ten times for one set. Rest for one to two minutes, then complete a second set of ten repetitions.

Tip: Be sure not to round or arch your back.

How Long Does It Take to Build Muscle?

Figure on a minimum of 12 to 15 weeks to build muscle, provided that you do 3 to 4 weight-training sessions per week. The typical workout is 6 to 15 repetitions—or sets—of about 8 to 12 different exercises.

How Much Muscle Can You Build?

Stick with the regimen and you can gain about 3 to 5 pounds of fat-free muscle mass, which burns more calories than fat.

SOURCE: David Nieman, Ph.D., Applachian State University, North Carolina

---

WEEK 5 GOALS

Monday	Tuesday	Wednesday	Thursday	Friday	Saturday	Sunday
☐	☐	☐	☐	☐	☐	☐

Record calories. Stay at the daily calorie level for your goals: _____

Fruit and vegetables (7–9 servings* per day)

☐☐☐☐☐ ☐☐☐☐☐ ☐☐☐☐☐ ☐☐☐☐☐ ☐☐☐☐☐ ☐☐☐☐☐ ☐☐☐☐☐
☐☐☐☐ ☐☐☐☐ ☐☐☐☐ ☐☐☐☐ ☐☐☐☐ ☐☐☐☐ ☐☐☐☐

*1 serving = 1 piece of fruit; 8 ounces of juice; ½ cup dried fruit; 1 cup cooked or raw vegetables; 2 cups raw, leafy greens (lettuce, spinach, arugula); 1 small potato

(continued)

Monday	Tuesday	Wednesday	Thursday	Friday	Saturday	Sunday

Fiber (25 grams a day for women and 38 grams a day for men 50 and younger; 21 grams per day for women and 30 grams per day for men 51 and older)

Your daily goal: _____

☐ ☐ ☐ ☐ ☐ ☐ ☐

Healthy fat (2 servings[†] per day).

☐☐ ☐☐ ☐☐ ☐☐ ☐☐ ☐☐ ☐☐

Protein (20–35 percent of daily calories: 100–175 grams on 2,000 calories per day)

☐ ☐ ☐ ☐ ☐ ☐ ☐

Eat healthy carbs (three 1-ounce servings daily of whole grains).

☐☐☐ ☐☐☐ ☐☐☐ ☐☐☐ ☐☐☐ ☐☐☐ ☐☐☐

Maintain 10 minutes more physical activity/day (beyond Week 1).

☐ ☐ ☐ ☐ ☐ ☐ ☐

Add resistance training (3 times weekly).   ☐   ☐   ☐

Reward _____ **Earned** ☐

SOURCES: 2005 Dietary Guidelines Advisory Committee Report; National Cancer Institute's 5 to 9 a Day program; National Academy of Sciences Dietary Reference Intakes

†A serving could be 2–3 ounces of fish or seafood (175–225 calories); 1/3 cup nuts (200 calories); 2 tablespoons of peanut butter (190 calories); 1/2 cup tofu (100 calories); 1/4 avocado (90 calories); 1 tablespoon of salad dressing made with canola, olive, safflower, or other healthy oil (80–120 calories); 1 tablespoon of Take Control or Benecol.

Eleven

WEEK 6: COUNT ON CALCIUM

In just a little over a month, you've already learned how to eat more of the fruits and vegetables that you enjoy best, not the ones that someone tells you to eat. You've also seen how to add healthy fat, boost protein, find the right caloric intake for your goals, choose healthy carbs, and add fiber—all important to feeling full and being well nourished. Plus, you've been moving more and learning how to make physical activity a daily habit. The resistance training that you added last week is one step toward building more muscle, which helps rev metabolism a little and also helps ensure healthier bones.

Boosting the essential mineral—calcium—is another important way to help preserve bone and prevent osteoporosis, a condition that affects 10 million Americans. Eighteen million more people have low bone mass, placing them at increased risk for osteoporosis, which results in fragile bones and increased risk of debilitating fractures.

A 2004 report from the U.S. surgeon general underscored why it's important not to skimp on dairy products when trying to whittle your waistline. Dairy products are rich in calcium, and many come fortified with vitamin D—a vitamin that a lot of Americans fall short on. Without enough vitamin D, calcium, and physical activity, it's hard to keep bones healthy.

As a result of these deficiencies, the report "Bone Health and

Osteoporosis" concludes that by 2020, one in two Americans over age 50 will be at risk for fractures or low bone mass related to osteoporosis.

Nor is this a problem only for older Americans. Janet Rubin, professor of medicine at Emory University, testified before Congress that military recruits are frequently deficient in both calcium and vitamin D. Due in part to poor bone health, as many as 5 percent of male recruits and up to 20 percent of female recruits suffer from stress fractures, Rubin reported.

Calcium does more than build strong bones, however. It also helps control blood pressure, aids in blood clotting, helps ensure nerve and muscle function, and may help reduce the risk of colon cancer or, at the very least, the recurrence of colon polyps. There's even tantalizing evidence that calcium may help control body weight. While the findings are still preliminary and very limited, a small, six-month study compared two groups trying to lose weight. Both ate the same number of calories, but one group took a dietary supplement with 800 milligrams of calcium daily. The other ate 1,200 to 1,300 milligrams daily of dairy products (about the amount found in three glasses of skim milk). People who ate the added dairy foods lost 70 percent more weight than those who took the dietary supplements.

Since more than a third of men and more than half of women don't get enough calcium daily, according to the USDA, calcium was dubbed a "shortfall nutrient" by the 2005 Dietary Guidelines Advisory Committee.

GOT MILK?

Dairy products are, of course, a prime source of calcium. But as the 2005 Dietary Guidelines Advisory Committee noted, "Many of the health benefits associated with milk consumption may be attributable" to other nutrients, including potassium, magnesium, and vitamins A and D. One USDA study of nearly 18,000 participants found that increasing milk consumption was linked with increased intakes of all micronutrients except for vitamin C. For those reasons, the committee recommended consumption of three cups of milk or milk products per day "to reduce the risk of low bone mass and contribute important amounts of many nutrients."

Calcium

What the experts say: adequate daily intake

19–50 years	1,000 milligrams
51+	1,200

How to get it in food: Eat about 2 cups of nonfat yogurt (total 900 milligrams) and drink a cup of skim milk (300 milligrams).

Don't exceed 2,500 milligrams.

SOURCES: National Academy of Sciences, Institute of Medicine, Dietary Reference Intakes, Calcium, Phosphorus, Magnesium, Vitamin D, and Fluoride; USDA; 2005 Dietary Guidelines Advisory Committee Report

---

If you're lactose intolerant or a vegetarian who doesn't eat dairy products, you may want to choose one of the many other calcium-rich options, including fortified juices, soy milk, cereal, bread, and snack bars and, of course, calcium supplements.

Here's how you can boost calcium daily for a variety of health benefits, including possibly a smaller waistline.

Get a smart start. A cup of nonfat yogurt or an ounce (about a cup) of fortified whole-grain cereal gets you at least halfway to the 1,000 daily milligrams of calcium considered adequate for those aged 19 to 50. Youngsters, teens, and pregnant or lactating women need 1,300 milligrams daily; adults 51 and older need 1,200 milligrams.

Both unsweetened cereal and nonfat, plain yogurt are caloric bargains. Depending on the brand, an ounce of fortified cereal packs 350 to 1,000 milligrams of calcium but has just 74 to 120 calories, according to the 2005 U.S. Dietary Guidelines Advisory Committee. A cup of plain nonfat yogurt has 127 calories but provides 452 milligrams of calcium. Add some fruit or a dab of honey for extra flavor. (See below why fruit is also good for bones.) One caveat: Yogurt is not usually fortified with vitamin D, as milk is.

Snack on seafood. Most fish and seafood are rich in vitamin D, which helps regulate blood levels of both calcium and phosphorus, important for strong bones. The higher the levels of vitamin D, the better the bone. An ounce of herring has 193 International Units (IU) of vitamin D, about the daily intake considered adequate by the National Academy of Sciences for healthy people aged 9 to 50. Older adults need twice that amount. A growing number of experts say that vitamin D recommendations are likely too low. Even so, women of childbearing age, as well as children, need to balance eating fish and seafood with concerns about mercury and other contaminants. So choose light tuna and limit consumption to no more than twice per week. Find more information at the Food and Drug Administration, www.cfsan.fda.gov/~dms/admehg3.html.

Leverage a calcium-rich beverage. Besides skim or 1 percent fat milk, options include soy milk or fruit juices fortified with calcium and vitamin D.

Color your plate. Here's yet another reason to eat more fruits and vegetables. Studies presented in recent years at the annual meeting of the American Society for Bone and Mineral Research suggest that fruits and vegetables alter blood acidity, which in turn helps minimize bone loss. So here's more motivation to get those recommended two cups a day of fruit and two and a half cups per day of vegetables.

Reach for leafy green vegetables. They're loaded with vitamin K. New research hints that vitamin K may boost production of a substance that helps preserve bone density. Spinach, kale, and broccoli also contain calcium, which is good for bones. But the calcium contained in vegetables is not as readily available to the bones as that from dairy products.

Toss some sesame seeds on your salad. An ounce of sesame seeds contains nearly the amount of calcium found in a glass of skim milk. But since it also has 160 calories—double the amount of the skim milk—you may need to make other caloric adjustments.

Lighten up on the java. Ditto for caffeinated soft drinks. In excess, caffeine is counterproductive to your calcium-boosting efforts. Excess caffeine is a minor risk factor for bone loss, because it helps promote calcium loss.

Hedge your bets with dietary supplements. Dairy products remain the leading source of calcium, but the American public falls chronically short of recommended daily goals. Scientists say that food is the optimal source of calcium and vitamin D, but if you're simply not getting enough servings of calcium- and vitamin D–rich food, then consider taking a calcium supplement to bridge the gap. Look for one with no more than 600 milligrams of calcium, since that's the most the body can absorb at one time. Choose a supplement that also includes vitamin D. Different types of calcium are absorbed in different ways. Calcium carbonate requires a little food for absorption; calcium citrate or malate can be taken on an empty stomach.

Chicago: Sally, the only surefire way for me to fit in my fitness is to do it really early in the morning (5:45 A.M.). My husband helps me get up by having a breakfast shake all made for me when I walk in the door after the workout. If I don't work out, I don't get breakfast. It's been a good motivator!

ALL SIZES FIT

Maintain resistance training three times a week and increase daily activity to 20 minutes above baseline. That takes you two-thirds of the way to the 30 minutes of daily physical activity recommended by the U.S. surgeon general. Of course, you can always do more. Not only does this activity help burn calories—roughly 80 per session, depending on body weight and intensity of the workout—but consistency helps to build strong exercise habits. Any activity that keeps you upright helps build and preserve bones. So walk, take the stairs, or just stand up frequently throughout the day. Jogging, step aerobics, and weight training also help improve bone health.

Alexandria, Va.: I have been to the holy land, and it is the free-weight room. After spending six months with a morning workout group and losing 30 pounds in the process, I felt like it was time to move on. Now I'm hitting the weights two to three times a week, along with cardio on the other days, and it's taken me to a whole new level. I'm starting to see abs even though I'm still at least 30 pounds overweight. My legs are decidedly thinner, even though I haven't lost more than a pound or two since I started lifting two weeks ago. So, my fellow women, hit those weights! And not the machines, except for a few cable exercises and the leg curls for those of us with weak hamstrings. Free weights make all of your dreams come true.

Sally Squires: Lifting weights is a great way to fight against the ravages of aging, since we all lose muscle with each advancing year, unless we take steps to thwart it. There's also good research from Tufts University to suggest that even 90-year-olds can benefit from weight training. So it's never too late to begin!

More activity has another advantage: It gives you a little wiggle room with calories. For example, just going from sedentary to moderate activity can make it possible to speed your efforts at achieving a healthy weight by burning more calories. Or it can give you a couple hundred calories more to eat without undermining your weight-loss efforts.

Sedentary means doing only the light physical activity associated with daily life, the equivalent of logging fewer than 7,000 steps per day on a pedometer. *Moderate* activity means walking 1½ to 3 miles per day at 15 to 20 minutes per mile. *Active* is walking at least 3 miles per day at 15 to 20 minutes per mile.

	Sedentary*	Moderately Active†	Active‡
Women Body mass index = 21.5; 31–50 years	1,800 calories/day	2,000 calories/day	2,200 calories/day
Men Body mass index = 22.5; 31–50 years	2,200 calories/day	2,400–2,600 calories/day	2,800–3,000 calories/day

SOURCE: 2005 Dietary Guidelines Advisory Committee Report, Section D, Table D3-1; Institute of Medicine, National Academy of Sciences

*Only light physical activity associated with daily life
†Walk 1½ to 3 miles daily at 3 to 4 mph or equivalent
‡Walk 3+ miles daily at 3 to 4 mph or equivalent

WEEK 6 GOALS

Monday   Tuesday   Wednesday   Thursday   Friday   Saturday   Sunday

Record calories. Stay at the daily calorie level for your goals: _____

☐   ☐   ☐   ☐   ☐   ☐   ☐

Fruit and vegetables (7–9 servings* per day)

☐☐☐☐☐   ☐☐☐☐☐   ☐☐☐☐☐   ☐☐☐☐☐   ☐☐☐☐☐   ☐☐☐☐☐   ☐☐☐☐☐
☐☐☐☐   ☐☐☐☐   ☐☐☐☐   ☐☐☐☐   ☐☐☐☐   ☐☐☐☐   ☐☐☐☐

*1 serving = 1 piece of fruit; 8 ounces of juice; ½ cup dried fruit; 1 cup cooked or raw vegetables; 2 cups raw, leafy greens (lettuce, spinach, arugula); 1 small potato

Fiber (25 grams a day for women and 38 grams a day for men 50 and younger; 21 grams per day for women and 30 grams per day for men 51 and older)

Your daily goal: _____

☐   ☐   ☐   ☐   ☐   ☐   ☐

Healthy fat (2 servings† per day).

☐☐   ☐☐   ☐☐   ☐☐   ☐☐   ☐☐   ☐☐

†A serving could be 2–3 ounces of fish or seafood (175–225 calories); ⅓ cup nuts (200 calories); 2 tablespoons of peanut butter (190 calories); ½ cup tofu (100 calories); ¼ avocado (90 calories); 1 tablespoon of salad dressing made with canola, olive, safflower, or other healthy oil (80–120 calories); 1 tablespoon of Take Control or Benecol.

Protein (20–35 percent of daily calories: 100–175 grams on 2,000 calories per day)

☐   ☐   ☐   ☐   ☐   ☐   ☐

Healthy carbs (three 1-ounce servings daily of whole grains)

☐☐☐   ☐☐☐   ☐☐☐   ☐☐☐   ☐☐☐   ☐☐☐   ☐☐☐

Add calcium (3 servings of milk or milk products daily).

☐☐☐   ☐☐☐   ☐☐☐   ☐☐☐   ☐☐☐   ☐☐☐   ☐☐☐

Monday	Tuesday	Wednesday	Thursday	Friday	Saturday	Sunday

Add 20 minutes more physical activity/day (beyond Week 1).

☐   ☐   ☐   ☐   ☐   ☐   ☐

Resistance training (3 times weekly).   ☐   ☐   ☐

Reward _____ **Earned**   ☐

SOURCES: 2005 Dietary Guidelines Advisory Committee Report; National Cancer Institute's 5 to 9 a Day program; National Academy of Sciences Dietary Reference Intakes

Twelve

WEEK 7: MINDFUL EATING

Now that you're beginning Week 7, you're already eating smart and moving more—two of the tenets of the Lean Plate Club. So you're well on the way to healthier habits.

Still, it may take more to reach your goals. With food readily available 24/7, there's temptation around every corner and likely within reach of you day and night. These days we can eat while walking down the street. We snack in front of the television, grab a bite in the car, gobble food at our desks, and munch midnight snacks while lying in bed. No wonder it's easy to be overnourished, even with healthful food. That's why it's important to track what you eat and to add more physical activity.

PORTION PATROL

The lament often goes like this: "I don't understand why I can't lose weight, because I'm eating all the right things."

Ah, but are you eating *too much* of the right things? Portion sizes are so distorted these days that it's easy to experience calorie creep without realizing it. You might think you're eating "hardly anything" when you're actually consuming a lot.

Even a few extra calories can add up big-time. Just 100 extra calories per day—about the amount found in half a single bag of potato chips—can pile on an extra ten pounds per year. That's why it's important not only to find the right caloric balance for your goals (as you did in Week 1) but also to make wise use of what the 2005 U.S. Dietary Guidelines Scientific Advisory Committee called "discretionary calories."

So what are discretionary calories?

They're the equivalent of a little loose change in your pocket— the difference between the calories needed to provide all the essential nutrients for health and the calories you burn daily. They're not just the icing on the cake—they are the cake *and* the icing. They're also the cream in whole milk, the added sugar in a soft drink, the fat in fried food, the margarine on your toast, and the dressing on your salad.

In other words, they're the high-calorie foods that appeal to your taste buds but pack minimal nutritional punch and often come loaded with calories that aren't helpful for your waistline— unless you happen to be very active every day.

The trouble is that many of us eat far too many discretionary calories, usually without realizing it. Here's how it shakes down: A typical 40-year-old sedentary office worker burns about 2,350 calories per day. He needs only 1,938 calories to meet his basic nutritional needs. So the difference—412 calories—is what he has left over for discretionary eating. He might use those calories to enjoy a beer and a small bag of potato chips while watching a Sunday afternoon football game on television. That is, if he limits himself to one beer and one small bag of chips.

Many of us engage in mindless eating—you know, a bag of chips here, a couple of cookies there, a treat at the office when a coworker brings in a cake, and then maybe there's a candy bar for the commute home.

It's just too easy to tip the balance the wrong way with discretionary calories. Studies show that the average overweight American underestimates daily caloric intake by up to 40 percent. On 2,000 calories a day—the typical amount recommended for many adults by the U.S. Dietary Guidelines—that works out to an extra 800 calories a day. Over a week, that adds up 5,600 calories, or about enough to pile on one and a half pounds per week.

What compounds the problem is that most people overestimate intake of healthful foods and underestimate consumption of unhealthful foods, according to studies at the University of Washington in Seattle. So if you're like most people, you probably think your diet is better than it really is.

HOW MANY DISCRETIONARY CALORIES CAN I HAVE?

That depends in part on your age and sex as well as the amount of physical activity you get each day. The more active you are, the greater your discretionary calorie allowance. By the same token, the less active you are, the fewer your discretionary calories. The numbers below show how small the wiggle room can be when you are sedentary.

	SEDENTARY*		ACTIVE†	
	Total daily calories	Discretionary calories	Total daily calories	Discretionary calories
Women				
19–30 years old	2,000	265	2,000–2,400	265–360
31–50	1,800	195	2,000–2,200	265–290
51+	1,600	130	1,800–2,200	195–290

| | SEDENTARY* | | ACTIVE† | |
	Total daily calories	Discretionary calories	Total daily calories	Discretionary calories
Men				
19–30 years old	2,400	360	2,600–3,000	410–510
31–50	2,200	290	2,400–3,000	360–510
51+	2,000	265	2,200–2,800	290–425

SOURCE: USDA, www.MyPyramid.gov

*You get less than 30 minutes daily of moderate exercise.
†You get between 30 and 60 minutes daily of moderate exercise.

Here's how you can engage in mindful eating and avoid portion distortion and calorie creep.

Rev up before coming to the table. That's right, instead of rushing to eat, do one to three minutes of brief exercise just before sitting down at the table. Take a brief walk, swing your arms to get the blood really moving, or find a stairwell and go up and down steps for one to two minutes before eating. Just a minute or two of exercise helps increase blood flow to the muscles and away from the stomach, which can help to temporarily decrease appetite. While it won't prevent gorging, it's an opportunity to stop and take account of what you are about to do.

Savor the flavor. Take the time to enjoy food. Focus on what you're consuming. Guilt—especially about eating so-called bad foods—fuels a lot of fast overeating. Give yourself permission to sit down and eat slowly. Better to savor two small chocolate chip cookies than to gobble ten without really tasting them and wind up feeling full and unsatisfied.

Divide and conquer. Take a serving of food. Give yourself half. Eat that. Then if you want to come back for seconds, have the other half. If not, you've cut your calories for that meal in half.

No standing meals. You know the drill. First you reach inside the fridge for one bite of something. Then it's another, and pretty soon you're sampling from all the leftovers. Without realizing it, you've eaten enough calories for a meal. Or maybe your favorite is standing over the kitchen sink to eat a fast meal. Go ahead, eat. Just make sure you do it sitting down—preferably not in front of the television.

Read Nutrition Labels

Will it make you a healthier eater? Maybe. Researchers at the Fred Hutchinson Cancer Institute in Seattle found that adults who read the nutrition facts box on food labels reduced their fat intake by 2 percent and slightly increased consumption of fruits and vegetables over a two-year period, compared to their non-label-reading peers.

SOURCES: Fred Hutchinson Cancer Institute; *Journal of the American Dietetic Association*

Always use utensils. When you grab a handful of this or a handful of that it's easy to lose track of how much you are eating. So put all food on a plate. Use utensils. They can help slow down your consumption.

Chewing counts. Yes, Mom was right when she said to chew slowly, but no, you don't have to chew everything 30 times. There's no evidence to suggest that it helps you decrease the amount of food you eat, but it may help make you more aware of what you're eating while you're eating it. Savor the flavor and texture of what you're eating. Practice enjoying—rather than quickly "inhaling"—your food.

Establish no-food zones. Eat at the kitchen or dining table, but not throughout the house and especially avoid eating while watching television. Establish no-food zones at the office and in the car.

Examine why you eat. The obvious question: Are you really hungry or are you eating for some other reason? Habit, boredom, stress, or just feeling out of control can fuel hunger. Eating is an easy way to keep emotions at bay—and unthinkingly sabotage your efforts.

Take a seventh-inning stretch. Postpone second helpings until at least ten minutes after finishing the first to enable your brain to catch up with the satiety signals from your stomach. Dish out single servings and keep platters in the kitchen rather than on the table, where they provide temptation. Be especially careful at restaurants, where serving sizes are often large. Split entrées or a couple of appetizers.

Water liberally during meals. Sip water between bites even if you're only snacking. The sodium in food helps you retain water. That, in turn, helps increase satiety and can help to slow consumption. Another tip: Put utensils down between mouthfuls just to slow down eating.

ALL SIZES FIT

Increase your daily physical activity to 25 minutes above Week 1. No need to engage in it all at once: The point is to make that activity a daily habit. By boosting time to 25 minutes daily, you're just five minutes short of the U.S. surgeon general's recommendation.

How much does that physical activity matter? Plenty. Emerging research suggests that many of the physical changes chalked up to growing old—insulin resistance, decreased lung function, and elevated systolic blood pressures—are not due to aging at all, but to inactivity. A 2002 *New England Journal of Medicine* study of more than 6,000 older men showed that poor physical fitness was a better predictor of premature death than smoking, hypertension, or heart disease.

That's why experts say that there's no drug in current or prospective use that holds as much promise for a life of extended vitality as does physical exercise. Plus, it's infinitely cheaper than buying medication. People who perform regular, vigorous workouts not only exhibit slower and smaller declines in aerobic capacity with advancing years but seem to hold the line on aging.

Not so for their less active counterparts. Beginning at middle age, aerobic capacity and muscle mass decrease about 10 percent per decade. And without regular exercise, physical decline doesn't just continue steadily; it accelerates beginning at about age 60—one more reason to make daily exercise a habit to offset that decline. And the good news is that it's never too late to start.

Stretch Your Limits

Not only will stretching help you feel good, but it's also good for your muscles, which shorten with age and inactivity. So one of this week's goals is also to add stretching to increase flexibility and keep muscles supple and toned.

Desk Sets

Contrary to popular wisdom and common practice, stretching before workouts does not help prevent injury or improve athletic performance. But where stretching seems to pay off with proven benefits is in the workplace.

Stretching helps counteract the muscle shortening that results from hours of sitting at a desk. It may also help reduce the risk of generalized aches and pains, cut the odds of developing blood clots in the legs, and decrease the risk of developing herniated disks in the back. (Since disks don't have their own blood supply, the only way to get them nourishment is to move them.)

That's where stretching comes in. (As always, if you have any health problems, check first with your doctor before doing any of these activities.) Stand every 60 to 90 minutes during the workday and do at least five stretches at your desk or cubicle.

- **Counteract desk hunching.** Stand with your arms hanging at your sides. Raise your arms straight out at shoulder level. Keep your elbows straight. Turn your palms up and point your thumbs back. Hold for five to ten counts. Repeat throughout the day.

- **Stop in the name of stretch!** Tapping a keyboard and using a mouse take a toll on your wrist flexors and extensors. That, in turn, can increase the chances of carpal tunnel syndrome and tennis and golfer's elbow. So standing or seated, put your right arm out in front of you, palm out like you're stopping traffic. Keep elbow straight. Use your left hand to gently pull the fingers of the right hand toward your face. Hold for about ten counts. Repeat with the other arm. Then, with both arms straight out in front of you, make fists and move your hands toward the floor to stretch your wrists. Hold for ten counts. If that's uncomfortable, start with five and gradually build up to ten. Relax briefly. Repeat.

- **Find your inner cat.** This helps nourish your vertebral disks. Stand. Bend your knees slightly, placing your hands just above your knees. Now arch your back gently up and then down like a cat. The middle of your back should move the most and, with it, all vertebrae.

- **Be hip.** Hip flexors often tighten with sitting. Stand. Place your left leg forward and your right leg back. Bend both knees slightly. Keep your feet flat. Move your hips slightly forward. Hold the position for ten counts, gradually increasing time to one minute. Repeat on the other side.

- **Tune your hamstrings.** Tight hamstrings are a common complaint of the desk bound. Stand and elevate your right leg on something stable that is about 12 to 16 inches high (a wastebasket or open desk drawer will do). If needed, place one hand on a wall, doorknob, or file cabinet for balance. Keep both knees slightly bent, especially the elevated knee. With your back straight, slowly lean forward until you feel a hamstring stretch at the back of the thigh. Stick out your derriere to stretch the hamstrings farther. Hold for ten counts. Repeat on the other side.

Hip Extension

The following exercises come from the National Institute on Aging. It's always a good idea to warm your muscles before stretching with walking, walking in place, or other gentle movement.

This hip-extension exercise helps to strengthen buttocks and lower-back muscles. Stand 12 to 18 inches from a table or chair, with your feet slightly apart. Holding on to the table or chair for balance, bend forward at the hips at about a 45-degree angle. Slowly lift one leg straight backward without bending your knee or arching your back. Point your toes. Tilt your upper body forward. Hold the position for one second. Slowly lower your leg. Pause. Repeat with the other leg. Alternate legs until you have done 8 to 15 repetitions with each leg. Rest, then do another set of 8 to 15 alternating repetitions. When you are ready, use ankle weights to increase intensity and build stronger muscles.

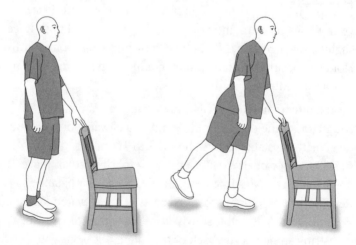

Hamstring Stretch

Sit sideways on a bench, on the floor, or another hard surface (such as two chairs placed side by side). Stretch one leg straight, toes pointed up. Keep your other leg off the bench with your foot flat on the floor, or to the side if you're on the floor. If your straight leg feels stretched, hold this position for 10 to 30 seconds. If you don't feel a stretch on the back of your leg, then lean forward from your hips (not your waist) until you feel a stretch in the back of your leg. Keep your back and shoulders straight. Hold for 10 to 30 seconds. Repeat with the other leg. Repeat three to five times on each side, breathing out as you stretch, very gently deepening the stretch. Don't bounce.

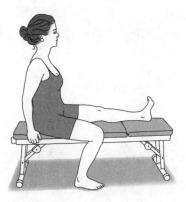

Alternative Hamstring Stretch

If you're really out of shape, it's important to proceed cautiously with all activities, including stretching, so as to minimize the risk of injuries that could sideline you and undermine your efforts. This alternative hamstring stretch also helps lengthen the muscles in the back of your thighs but does it from a standing position. Get a straight-backed chair. Hold the back with both hands and move your feet back so that when you bend forward from your hips, your back and shoulders are straight. Keep your back and shoulders straight at all times. When your upper body is parallel to the floor, hold your position for 10 to 30 seconds. You should feel a stretch in the back of your thighs. Be sure not to bounce. Repeat three to five times.

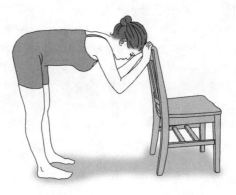

Quadriceps Stretch

Lie on your side with your head on a pillow or on your hand. Keep your hips in a straight line, one directly above the other. Bend the knee that is on top. Reach back and grab your heel with your top hand. If you can't reach it, loop a towel or belt over your foot or ankle. Gently pull your leg until you feel a stretch in the front of your thigh. Hold the position for 10 to 30 seconds. Reverse the position and repeat. Repeat three to five times on each side. If the back of your thigh cramps during this exercise, stretch your leg and try again, but more slowly.

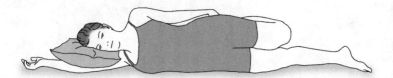

Calf Stretch

This helps stretch lower leg muscles. Stand with your hands against the wall, arms outstretched and elbows straight. Keep your left knee slightly bent, the toes of your right foot slightly turned inward. Step back one to two feet from the wall with your right leg, heel and foot remaining flat on the floor. You should feel a gentle stretch in your calf muscle. Don't bounce. If you don't feel a stretch, move your foot farther back until you do. Hold the position for 10 to 30 seconds. Bend your right knee, keeping the heel and foot flat on the floor. Hold the position for another 10 to 30 seconds. Repeat with your left leg. Repeat three to five times for each leg.

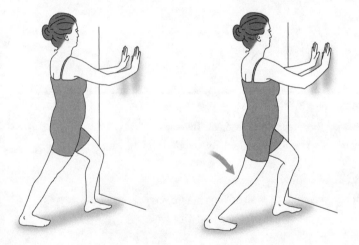

Triceps Stretch

Get a towel. Hold one end of the towel in your right hand. Raise and bend your right arm to drape the towel down your back. Keep your right arm in this position and continue holding on to the towel. Reach behind your lower back and grasp the bottom end of towel with your left hand. Climb your left hand progressively higher up the towel, which pulls your right arm down. Continue

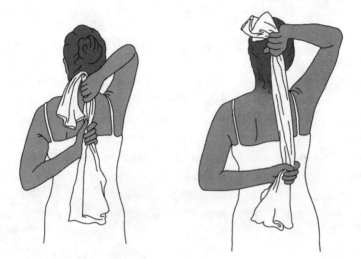

until your hands touch, or as close to that as you can comfortably go. Reverse positions. Repeat each position three to five times.

WEEK 7 GOALS

| Monday | Tuesday | Wednesday | Thursday | Friday | Saturday | Sunday |

Record calories. Stay at the daily calorie level for your goals: _____

☐   ☐   ☐   ☐   ☐   ☐   ☐

Fruit and vegetables (7–9 servings* per day)

Fruit _____ cups*/daily for your calorie level

☐   ☐   ☐   ☐   ☐   ☐   ☐

Vegetables _____ cups*/daily for your calorie level

☐   ☐   ☐   ☐   ☐   ☐   ☐

*1 serving = 1 piece of fruit; 8 ounces of juice; ½ cup dried fruit; 1 cup cooked or raw vegetables; 2 cups raw, leafy greens (lettuce, spinach, arugula); 1 small potato

Fiber (25 grams a day for women and 38 grams a day for men 50 and younger; 21 grams per day for women and 30 grams per day for men 51 and older)

Monday	Tuesday	Wednesday	Thursday	Friday	Saturday	Sunday

Your daily goal:

☐ ☐ ☐ ☐ ☐ ☐ ☐

Healthy fat (2 servings† per day)

☐☐ ☐☐ ☐☐ ☐☐ ☐☐ ☐☐ ☐☐

†A serving could be 2–3 ounces of fish or seafood (175–225 calories); ⅓ cup nuts (200 calories); 2 tablespoons of peanut butter (190 calories); ½ cup tofu (100 calories); ¼ avocado (90 calories); 1 tablespoon of salad dressing made with canola, olive, safflower, or other healthy oil (80–120 calories); 1 tablespoon of Take Control or Benecol.

Protein (20–35 percent of daily calories: 100–175 grams on 2,000 calories per day)

☐ ☐ ☐ ☐ ☐ ☐ ☐

Healthy carbs (three 1-ounce servings daily of whole grains).

☐☐☐ ☐☐☐ ☐☐☐ ☐☐☐ ☐☐☐ ☐☐☐ ☐☐☐

Calcium (3 servings of milk or milk products daily).

☐☐☐ ☐☐☐ ☐☐☐ ☐☐☐ ☐☐☐ ☐☐☐ ☐☐☐

Engage in mindful eating.

☐☐☐ ☐☐☐ ☐☐☐ ☐☐☐ ☐☐☐ ☐☐☐ ☐☐☐

Add 25 minutes more physical activity/day (beyond Week 1).

☐ ☐ ☐ ☐ ☐ ☐ ☐

Resistance training (3 times weekly)   ☐   ☐   ☐

Stretch (3 times weekly).   ☐   ☐   ☐

Reward _____ **Earned** ☐

SOURCES: 2005 Dietary Guidelines Advisory Committee Report; National Cancer Institute's 5 to 9 a Day program; National Academy of Sciences Dietary Reference Intakes

Thirteen

WEEK 8: SLEEP TO REACH YOUR DREAMS

To sleep, perchance to dream . . .
—*William Shakespeare,* Hamlet

Seven weeks ago, you began a journey toward healthier habits. Now you know how to make smart choices to eat a varied diet filled with the healthful, great-tasting foods that you like best—not the ones that someone tells you to consume. You're aware of portion distortion and calorie creep, and know how to find your own caloric balance. You know that fat is not a four-letter word and can tell the difference between healthy fat and saturated and trans fats, which help to increase the risk of heart disease. You know the importance of getting enough protein to feel full and understand that choosing whole-grain foods over highly processed fare will help keep your blood sugar and insulin levels steady and enable you to avoid the rapid cycling of ravenous hunger followed by overeating.

You're also getting 25 minutes more physical activity per day than when you started. That alone puts you in a new league of your own.

Now comes the fine-tuning, because what you're doing is great, but it's just the beginning of the rest of your life. This is where changing habits parts company from dieting, which by its very nature is for a limited period of time. As you continue to get into a good rhythm with eating smart and moving more throughout the day, it's time to take a look at how other things affect how hungry you feel, how much energy you have, and, yes, may even undermine your efforts.

CONTROL YOUR APPETITE WITH Z'S

Sleep is one of the first items shortchanged in this busy, harried life. For that reason, one of this week's goals is to get eight hours of sleep nightly.

No, that goal isn't a guess or a reflection of conventional wisdom. It's based on years of research that suggest adults need an average of eight to eight and a half hours of sleep each night—about an hour more than most of us typically get, according to the National Sleep Foundation.

Aside from being chronically sleep deprived—and often grumpy—there's growing evidence to suggest that lack of sleep wreaks havoc with appetite, insulin levels, and blood sugar. At the University of Chicago, sleep researcher Eve Van Cauter, Ph.D., and her colleagues took a group of lean, healthy young men and put them in a sleep lab for 16 nights. After letting them sleep normally for a few days, the researchers deprived the volunteers of a couple of hours of sleep each night and then gave them a battery of blood tests.

The results showed significant changes in levels of leptin and cortisol, two key hormones that regulate hunger. Sleep loss stimulated appetite. It was as if the participants' bodies were screaming "starvation" despite the fact that they didn't physiologically need to eat. Participants responded by increasing food as if they were missing about 1,000 calories a day. You can imagine how many pounds that would add if they were allowed to continue.

The sleep disruption also pushed these young men into a prediabetic state called impaired glucose tolerance, a condition that now afflicts millions of overweight and obese adults worldwide. By losing just a few hours of sleep per night, these young, healthy study participants developed insulin and blood sugar levels that suddenly resembled those of adults 65 to 80 years old. Fortunately, the study participants' blood chemistry, and hunger, returned to normal after they got enough sleep.

In a follow-up study, the same team of researchers tested healthy men and women with an average body mass index of 23, considered well within the range for healthy body weight. Half the group were normal sleepers, getting 7½ to 8½ hours per night. The other half were short sleepers, who averaged 6½ hours or less.

Glucose tolerance tests showed that the short sleepers were experiencing hormonal changes that could affect their future body weight and impair their long-term health. To keep their blood sugar levels normal, the short sleepers needed to make 30 percent more insulin than the normal sleepers. Even though they weren't yet overweight, their profiles predisposed them to put on weight.

Another tantalizing clue about the impact of sleep loss on appetite and body weight comes from studies of people with sleep apnea. Those whose sleep is interrupted by apnea—brief episodes when breathing stops—have impaired glucose tolerance compared with folks the same weight without apnea.

Some of the most intriguing evidence for the link between sleep loss and weight gain comes from the obesity epidemic itself. Increased food consumption and decreased physical activity have certainly powered the nation's increase in girth. But researchers agree that those two things alone can't explain the entire obesity epidemic.

What else has changed? You guessed it: sleep. The average amount of nightly sleep for adults in the United States has declined by about one and a half hours during the past two decades. Match that against the rise in obesity, and a mirror image occurs. That suggests, according to Van Cauter and others, that sleep loss may be an important risk factor for obesity.

More recent findings back that up. The Wisconsin Sleep Cohort Study involving 1,024 participants found a link between amount of sleep and body mass index. Those who slept fewer than eight hours had higher body mass indexes and altered hormone levels of leptin and ghrelin, two key hormones that regulate appetite.

So how do you fit more sleep into a busy schedule?

Make sleep a priority. The average adult is chronically sleep deprived. It's easy to give sleep short shrift, but you really do need eight hours nightly. So if you stay up late one night, make up the lost sleep within a few days either by sleeping later, going to bed earlier, or napping.

Rule out any medical problems. Allergies, a deviated septum, infections, sleep apnea, and a condition called restless legs can all interfere with getting enough z's. Seek treatment for these problems, including nasal sprays and antihistamines that can help prevent nighttime nasal congestion. Mouth guards can help with teeth grinding. There's a C-Pap device to treat apnea, and nasal strips can help reduce snoring. Prescription medication is available to help reduce restless leg syndrome and a condition called myoclonus—full-body contractions that can jerk you awake.

Take your bedroom's temperature. Premenopausal and postmenopausal women can have hot flashes that interrupt sleep. Adjust bedroom temperature and bedding accordingly. Check out some of the new pillows or pads that can go into the freezer or come filled with coolants. When placed underneath your head or body, they can help to make you feel cooler. Fans near the bed can also help keep things cool, no matter what time of year.

Mute the noise level. Nix falling asleep in front of the television. When you wake up and go to bed, it's often hard to get back to sleep. Try reading or listening to soothing music instead. Consider a white noise machine to drown out environmental noise, or simply get a small fan.

Skip alcohol and cut back on caffeine in the hours before

bedtime. Alcohol initially promotes sleep but then seems to interrupt it, the reason that many people nod off after having a drink or two and then find themselves wide awake in bed, staring at the ceiling a few hours later. Sensitivity to caffeine varies widely. But many people find that, particularly as they age, they need to stop drinking caffeinated beverages after noon unless their goal is to stay up late. Decaffeinated coffee and tea are options, but still contain small amounts of caffeine that may be enough to keep awake those very sensitive to caffeine's effects.

Practice good sleep habits. Establish a regular sleep routine. Go to bed at roughly the same time every night, even on weekends. Wake up at about the same time every morning. Keep your bedroom solely for sleeping. Turn off the television, video games, and stereo. Avoid spending time in front of the computer for the hour or two before bedtime. There's some suggestion that the light could help confuse your biological clock. And when you have trouble getting to sleep, take long, slow cleansing breaths and practice progressive relaxation. Mentally think of each part of your body and imagine it relaxing. Work from your head to your toes.

Take a hot shower or bath about an hour before bedtime. Doing so raises your core body temperature. As it drops back to normal, it can help you fall into a deep sleep.

ALL SIZES FIT

Boost your daily physical activity to 30 minutes above what you were doing on Week 1. That takes you to the daily level recommended by the U.S. surgeon general.

Discovering new ways to be physically active throughout the day is an important key to long-term success for Lean Plate Club members. Steven N. Blair, Ph.D., president and CEO of the Cooper Institute, an internationally known exercise research center in Dallas, and exercise expert notes that the increased use of the computer, longer commutes to work, and a host of labor-saving devices all conspire to engineer physical activity out of our daily lives. That's just another reason to keep searching for enjoyable, inviting ways to boost your daily exercise.

Just make sure that as you become more active, you don't make the mistake of eating too many extra calories. Scientists have long debated whether exercise helps fuel appetite.

Numerous studies suggest that moderate- to high-intensity aerobic exercise—such as brisk walking, jogging, rowing, or cycling—has no impact on appetite in men. But a study by University of Ottawa researchers paints a different picture for women.

The researchers compared the effects of easy workouts and high-intensity exercise on appetite in 13 fit, lean women in their twenties. After each morning exercise session, the women had lunch at a buffet where they could eat as much as they wanted. They also had access to unlimited snacks and dined at the buffet in the evening.

High-intensity workouts—jogging at a fast pace, for example—greatly fueled appetite. After these sessions, women in the study ate enough food throughout the day to equal about 90 percent of the calories that they had burned by exercising. Much of the extra calories also came from high-fat food. Even after lower-intensity activities—for example, brisk walking—the women still ate about 35 percent of the calories that they had burned while exercising.

The researchers, who published their findings in the *American Journal of Clinical Nutrition,* advised women to be aware that exercise, particularly high-intensity activity, could significantly boost their appetites. These results could also help explain why men in weight-loss programs often seem to find more appetite control from exercise than women do. For example, in the Midwest Exercise Trial, a 16-month study of 131 overweight young adults who simply added physical activity to their daily regimen but didn't change what they ate, men lost an average of 11 pounds while women maintained their weight.

Here are some other tips to keep in mind about the effects of exercise on your appetite.

Physical activity always beats sedentary living. At the University of Ottawa, researchers also included a control session of no activity, after which they tracked what participants ate. Women consumed more net calories after being inactive for the morning than when they worked out intensively or moderately.

Skip snacks right after workouts. You may feel that you deserve an energy bar or a sports drink for your efforts, but if you're trying to trim pounds, adding calories in the two hours after workouts can be counterproductive. Doing so short-circuits fat burning and can undercut what you have done during exercise. So try to quench your thirst with water. And if you must eat soon after a workout, avoid food that raises blood sugar and results in a burst of insulin. Smart choices: a piece of fruit or a glass of vegetable juice.

Expect only modest calorie burn from exercise. It may feel like you burned a ton of calories in your step aerobics class, but odds are you didn't burn as many as you think. A 140-pound person who walks 1½ miles in 30 minutes burns roughly 100 calories—about the amount found in a medium chocolate chip cookie. So try to be realistic about how many calories you've really burned during a workout. And don't rely on the machines at the gym for an accurate count of your calories burned. They often are very inaccurate.

Stick with it. A yearlong study at the University of Pittsburgh found that adding regular physical activity produced weight loss in 200 overweight, sedentary women who were also dieting. Those who worked out about 20 minutes daily achieved a 7-pound weight loss, about a 5 percent weight reduction for someone who weighs 150 pounds. Women who spent 30 minutes daily exercising achieved more than twice that, equal to losing about 20 pounds for someone who weighs 150 pounds.

Plus, exercise delivers benefits that go far beyond trimming pounds or maintaining weight, including increased energy, better cardiovascular health, reduced stress, improved sleep, and better mood. Bottom line: Being active helps decrease blood flow to the stomach and opens it up to the muscles and heart, which is the exact opposite of what happens when you sit in front of the television and eat food.

WEEK 8 GOALS

Monday	Tuesday	Wednesday	Thursday	Friday	Saturday	Sunday

Record calories. Stay at the daily calorie level for your goals: _____

☐   ☐   ☐   ☐   ☐   ☐   ☐

Fruit and vegetables (7–9 servings* per day)

☐☐☐☐☐ ☐☐☐☐☐ ☐☐☐☐☐ ☐☐☐☐☐ ☐☐☐☐☐ ☐☐☐☐☐ ☐☐☐☐☐
☐☐☐☐   ☐☐☐☐   ☐☐☐☐   ☐☐☐☐   ☐☐☐☐   ☐☐☐☐   ☐☐☐☐

*1 serving = 1 piece of fruit; 8 ounces of juice; ½ cup dried fruit; 1 cup cooked or raw vegetables; 2 cups raw, leafy greens (lettuce, spinach, arugula); 1 small potato

Fiber (25 grams a day for women and 38 grams a day for men 50 and younger; 21 grams per day for women and 30 grams per day for men 51 and older)

Your daily goal: _____

☐   ☐   ☐   ☐   ☐   ☐   ☐

Healthy fat (2 servings[†] per day)

☐☐   ☐☐   ☐☐   ☐☐   ☐☐   ☐☐   ☐☐

†A serving could be 2–3 ounces of fish or seafood (175–225 calories); ⅓ cup nuts (200 calories); 2 tablespoons of peanut butter (190 calories); ½ cup tofu (100 calories); ¼ avocado (90 calories); 1 tablespoon of salad dressing made with canola, olive, safflower, or other healthy oil (80–120 calories); 1 tablespoon of Take Control or Benecol.

(continued)

Monday   Tuesday   Wednesday   Thursday   Friday   Saturday   Sunday

Protein (20–35 percent of daily calories: 100–175 grams on 2,000 calories per day)

☐   ☐   ☐   ☐   ☐   ☐   ☐

Healthy carbs (three 1-ounce servings daily of whole grains)

☐☐☐ ☐☐☐   ☐☐☐   ☐☐☐   ☐☐☐   ☐☐☐   ☐☐☐

Calcium (3 servings of milk or milk products daily)

☐☐☐ ☐☐☐   ☐☐☐   ☐☐☐   ☐☐☐   ☐☐☐   ☐☐☐

Mindful eating

☐☐☐ ☐☐☐   ☐☐☐   ☐☐☐   ☐☐☐   ☐☐☐   ☐☐☐

Add 30 minutes more physical activity/day (beyond Week 1).

☐   ☐   ☐   ☐   ☐   ☐   ☐

Resistance training (3 times weekly)   ☐   ☐   ☐

Stretch (3 times weekly).   ☐   ☐   ☐

Sleep 8 hours/night.

☐   ☐   ☐   ☐   ☐   ☐   ☐

Reward _____ **Earned** ☐

SOURCES: 2005 Dietary Guidelines Advisory Committee Report; National Cancer Institute's 5 to 9 a Day program; National Academy of Sciences Dietary Reference Intakes; Eve Van Cauter, Ph.D., University of Chicago

Part Three

HEALTHY HABITS FOR LIFE

Fourteen

SUCCESSFUL LOSERS

Congratulations! You've finished the Lean Plate Club eight-week program. This is just the beginning of your new healthy habits. If you had only a few pounds to lose to reach a healthier weight, you may have already reached your goal. But if you go back to your old habits, odds are the weight will return, too. For those who have more pounds to trim to achieve a healthier weight, you've got more time to practice those healthy habits to get to where you want to be. Behavioral research suggests that it takes about six months to really instill a healthy new habit.

New York: Hi, Sally! Regarding success strategies—the one time I was able to lose a lot of weight (30 pounds) and keep it off for a while was when my roommates and I all did the same program together and were each other's support group. I think that kind of support (and lack of temptation) helps with individual success.

The truth is that losing weight is just one part of a healthier lifestyle. Maintaining that weight loss is where the rubber hits the road. But there's good news to report. It appears that with time, weight maintenance gets easier.

Often lost amid the gloomy reports about the obesity epidemic is the fact that there are a growing number of successful losers—

people who not only lose pounds but manage to maintain their healthier weight long-term. Successful losers are of great interest to scientists, who see promise in their experience and lessons for others.

In fact, successful losers are so intriguing to researchers that Rena Wing, Ph.D., professor of psychiatry and behavior at Brown University, and James O. Hill, Ph.D., director of the Center for Human Nutrition at the University of Colorado Health Sciences Center, have teamed together to form a national database of successful losers. Known as the National Weight Control Registry, it includes more than 4,000 people—among them, a number of Lean Plate Club members—who have lost an average of 70 pounds and kept it off for more than five years. (To be eligible for the registry, you need to have lost at least 30 pounds and kept it off for at least a year.)

One of the biggest surprises from the National Weight Control Registry is that with time, weight maintenance gets easier. People who maintained their new weight for two years had a greater likelihood of keeping it off for two more years. Those who maintained it for five years increased the odds of maintaining their current weight even longer.

But weight maintenance doesn't happen automatically. It takes the same focus, commitment, and attention to detail that successful weight loss involves, as many Lean Plate Club successful losers will tell you. That's another reason why gradually achieving a healthier weight can set the foundation for your new thinner life.

Here's what Lean Plate Club successful losers advise.

Don't expect a quick fix. Nutrition fads come and go. It would be wonderful if one day scientists could report a foolproof, safe way to quickly drop unwanted pounds. But it doesn't exist now and it doesn't appear that there's anything like that in any research pipeline.

Successful losers report reaching a healthier weight the old-fashioned way: They count calories, reduce calorie-dense food, and move a lot more. About half of them report losing weight entirely on their own—no doctor, no special diet, no group meetings. The other half find assistance from commercial weight-loss programs, a physician, or a registered dietician. "Over the years, I tried a lot of different things—Jenny Craig, Weight Watchers a couple of times, different combinations of diets in magazines," said Melissa Glassman, a lawyer from northern Virginia who has shed half her body weight since joining the Lean Plate Club. "I could always lose 10 to 20 pounds but would always gain back more than that."

It was only by changing her habits that Melissa finally trimmed her weight from 250 to 125 pounds in a couple of years. She achieved and has maintained that loss with small steps that have added up to big rewards. "It's the little things that you incorporate into your daily life that help keep you on track," she said. "It doesn't have to be entirely about deprivation or exercising two hours a day."

Successful losers stay active by walking and

Weight lifting	20 percent
Riding a bike	20 percent
Aerobic exercise	18 percent

SOURCE: National Weight Control Registry

Find ways to be active throughout the day. It's possible to lose weight by simply eating less. But only about one in ten successful losers uses that approach. The majority—87 percent—eat fewer calories *and* burn more calories by becoming more physically active every day. They spend at least an hour a day doing something physical, whether it's walking briskly (about three to four miles per hour), taking the stairs whenever possible, walking or riding to errands, or commuting to work by bike or foot. Some who live great distances from their offices get off the subway or bus a few stops early and hoof it the rest of the way to their jobs.

It was just that activity that has helped one 45-year-old Lean Plate Club member from northern Virginia lose 156 pounds since 2001. Walking is the only activity that this federal worker does to keep in shape and maintain her impressive weight loss. She is motivated by her "coach," an active, high-energy dog she adopted from the animal shelter. "If we don't go for two walks a day, she's annoying. So we go for about two miles in the morning and about a mile at night."

Regular constitutionals have also helped another middle-aged Lean Plate Club member lose more than 100 pounds during the past two years. Like many people, this man is a "desk jockey" who spends a lot of time sitting during the day. Only by walking a couple of hours daily did he start to really see progress with his weight. He gets up early to make time for walking before work and family take over. The result: He's trimmed down to about 260 pounds from an all-time high of more than 400 pounds. As he puts it: "I have the same twenty-four hours in the day as everyone else." What counts for him is making exercise a priority—a change echoed by other successful Lean Plate Club members.

Track your weight. Nearly half of successful losers weigh themselves daily. "The scale is just a number to me now," said a Canadian Lean Plate Club member who has lost 140 pounds from her peak weight of 315 pounds. Regular weigh-ins have taught this LPCer that her weight naturally fluctuates by a couple of pounds either way. Getting on the scale "doesn't make or break my day," she said.

Enlist support. One Lean Plate Club successful loser who lives on the East Coast teamed with a relative in Texas to lose weight. Both joined Weight Watchers groups, then used phone calls and e-mails to encourage each other's efforts. Deborah Kosnett of Gaithersburg, Maryland, found support from her husband, who bought her a "comfort" bike with a wider seat and extra shock absorption and started her on a ride to a healthier life. Today, she's 85 pounds leaner and has pedaled well past that comfort bike to a sleek racing bike.

Some find that joining a group helps. Lean Plate Club member Melissa Glassman spends so much of her workday sitting that she joined an exercise group. In that way, she was able to find companionship and support as she strengthened her core muscles and lifted weights. "Part of my success is that I built a lot more muscle mass than I had before," she said, "and that made a big difference" in burning calories.

Start your day with breakfast. Almost 80 percent of successful losers eat a morning meal daily. The typical breakfast: cereal with skim milk and fruit. Make it whole-grain, unsweetened cereal for more staying power until lunch without hunger pangs.

Set small goals. Most people think too big and then feel very disheartened when they fall short of their goals. Losing at least 30 percent of their body weight is a commonly shared goal among overweight people. Yet from a medical standpoint, trimming just 10 percent of pounds—that's 20 pounds for someone who weighs 200 pounds—can have huge health benefits. So rather than set yourself up for failure—and possible yo-yo dieting—establish a more reasonable goal. Once you achieve that, then try for more. But take it step by step.

Find a good reason to get started. Reaching their all-time peak weight is what about 21 percent of successful losers say finally prompted them to get focused on achieving a healthier weight. But the most common trigger was a medical event—for example, a doctor's advice to lose weight, diagnosis of a condition such as high blood pressure, or a family member's heart attack. "My health was going bad," noted Kosnett. "I had prediabetes. My total blood cholesterol was not so great. It went as high as 260. My HDL (the 'good' cholesterol) was really lousy. But the straw that broke the camel's back was when I went out to sweep my front porch and I started panting. I thought, 'This is really stupid.'"

Set a limit for regaining pounds. If you reach it, switch from weight maintenance back to weight loss. Successful losers still experience slips but appear to be better than others at identifying them and making quick course corrections. Studies show that once you start to regain weight, if you put on more than ten pounds, then your chances of recovery are slim. "Every day, I have to stay on top of this," said Melissa Glassman.

Have a plan—and a backup strategy. Glassman eats only at restaurants where she knows the menu and can find something healthy to order. Each Monday, one Lean Plate Club successful loser stocks a week's worth of food in a freezer at her office to microwave for lunch each day.

When Deborah Kosnett required back surgery last year, she took precautions to maintain her weight. Knowing that she wouldn't be able to work out and would require prednisone, a powerful steroid that often adds weight, Deborah reduced her daily calories and carefully recorded what she ate. She also added more high-volume food—especially fruit—to combat hunger. The result? She lost five pounds during her convalescence and achieved her Weight Watchers goal weight.

Prepare psychologically for plateaus. Even when you do all the right things, it's usual for weight loss to slow, stabilize, or even reverse a little bit for brief periods of time. Deborah Kosnett experienced a plateau that lasted for a year and a half. A Canadian Lean Plate Club member had already lost 70 pounds when she hit her first plateau, which lasted four months. Although initially discouraged, she said she felt better when she realized that "it was awesome to maintain this huge weight loss." Her second plateau occurred after she had lost 100 pounds. "I couldn't get upset by it," she said. "My body had to get used to the new way of eating, the intensifying activity. We are not robots."

Don't forget to reward yourself. Behavioral research shows that this is key for long-term success—provided that you reach your preset goals. Some Lean Plate Club successful losers give themselves nonfood rewards such as having a pedicure, massage, facial, or manicure. You could buy yourself a favorite movie on DVD, get a book or CD that you've been longing for, or treat yourself to a new pair of workout shoes or a lesson with a pro. As she slowly but steadily transformed her body, Melissa Glassman bought new clothes at a discount store so she didn't wind up with an expensive wardrobe that was unusable. "I didn't want to spend a lot of money, because I was still in the process of losing weight," she said.

Stick with it for the long haul. Successful losers don't stop their healthy habits when they reach their goal weights. They commit for the long term. "I know that if I use the habits and the information that I've learned, I will be okay," said one Lean Plate Club successful loser. "I truly feel for the first time that my weight is under control."

And so can yours. By using the healthy habits that you have learned to think and act and eat and move like a thinner person, you increase the odds that you will achieve your goals. For life.

HOW TO KEEP SLIPS FROM BECOMING SLIDES INTO FAILURE

Call it slipping, stumbling, burnout, or simply boredom. Odds are that sooner or later, the glow you feel now about eating healthfully and being physically active wears off. Your weight plateaus. Fewer people comment on your changed appearance. You're not feeling your clothes getting looser. Suddenly, you may find that it's not quite as exciting to get up early to work out, to find time to take a walk at lunch, or even to pack a healthy lunch.

If you think this won't happen to you, think again. Still don't believe me? Then wait to read this section until you do experience a serious case of nutritional mischief or a bout of extended physical inertia.

Trust me. You'll be back. Studies suggest that nearly everyone who is serious about changing his or her habits eventually slips up. Call it bad habit quicksand. Once you step in it, you start to sink. This kind of diet fatigue is so common that some university-based weight-loss clinics warn their patients about it before it happens. Most shrug off the alerts. Some even get annoyed until it happens to them. But sooner or later, pretty much everyone hits the wall of healthy living.

The signs are small and insidious. "I find it harder to stay motivated" is the way one Lean Plate Club member, who had lost 60 pounds over a year and a half, described it. "I am feeling the pounds creep back, yet I can't seem to do anything about it. I have no ambition to get on the treadmill or go for a bike ride anymore and I don't even have an excuse like being too busy. I just simply don't want to. What's happening to me? I've worked so hard to achieve this weight loss, I just don't understand it. I'm so worried I'm going to be fat again. I can't get seem to get back to the mind-set I was in during my most motivated time. Help me so I don't gain it all back!"

Here's what can help you get back on track.

Pacific Northwest.: Holidays are tough for me, but I've found that one of the easier ways for me to survive them without blowing my diet is to give myself permission to take a taste of anything I want. If the item isn't part of a meal, then all I get is one small taste. This is enough for me to say, "Oh, this is just marvelous!" while usually thinking "too salty, too greasy, not really tasty, and not worth the calories." This year, I also hung a small mirror on my freezer door. I want to preserve my current look, so the mirror helps a lot.

Look at the big picture. Think of what you're doing not as a 100-yard dash but as a marathon or as the Tour de France. You're in it for the long haul. Changing habits takes time and commitment. Most people don't allow enough of either. Figure on a minimum of six months to instill healthier habits.

Cambridge, Mass.: I lowered my "watch-out" weight number to two pounds over my usual weight. At that weight, I go strictly back to fruits, vegetables, whole grains, milk, exercise, and water. When I'm back to normal, then I can start eating a few more indulgences.

Keep your habits fresh. If your morning workouts are feeling, well, too routine, try a workout at lunch or at night. When you can't bear to eat oatmeal another morning for breakfast, switch to egg-white omelets or whole-grain waffles or yogurt with fruit or even low-fat pizza made with whole-grain pita bread and nonfat or low-fat cheese.

When you begin to dread going to your step aerobics class, try spinning or cycling, yoga, Pilates, or tai chi. Add new healthy foods regularly. (In fact, on the weekly Lean Plate Club Web chat, prizes are awarded each week to a handful of Lean Plate Club members for coming up with clever, healthy food finds. Share some of yours at www.washingtonpost.com/leanplateclub from 1 to 2 P.M. EST Tuesdays. If you don't have time to join the chat live,

---

Rockville, Md.: My biggest challenges are buffets and potlucks—I feel like I need to have something of everything. Even if the portions are relatively small, if there are lots of good things to try, it's still too much food. When I thought about it a bit, I realized I feel an obligation to "honor" each different food by eating it—as if the food cared! Now hopefully I can laugh at my silliness and break the habit.

---

you can leave your suggestions or tips ahead of time and then come back later and read the transcript.) Or e-mail me anytime at leanplateclub@washpost.com. I read all my e-mail and answer as many messages as time permits.

Silver Spring, Md.: In order not to eat too much at parties or dinners, I make a bag of 94 percent fat-free microwave popcorn about an hour before I leave and eat half of the bag and drink a few glasses of water. I find it really fills me up and I don't feel like I need to eat the hors d'oeuvres or chips and dips while waiting for dinner. I also feel full enough to have smaller portions. And I make sure to get some club soda or sparkling water right away if it is a "bar" type party or to keep my water glass full if it is a sit-down meal.

Relax a little. Find small ways to loosen up, not quit, your healthy habits. If you've been religiously recording every morsel that passes your lips and can't bear the thought of writing down another entry, then note what you eat every other day for a while. (But don't use that as an excuse to go wild with food, either.) Or just record your food for a while on weekends. Or just after 3 P.M., if nighttime eating is a problem. In other words, give yourself a little break that doesn't let you stray too far from your usual pattern.

Draw a red line. Decide now that if your weight goes 2 or 5 or 10 pounds above where you are now, you'll immediately reinstate your full spectrum of habits that enabled you to achieve a healthier weight. If you reach that level, put your plan into action right away so that no more damage occurs.

Denver, Colo.: I've been keeping a food diary in an Excel spreadsheet I made for myself. It's really great to get a running total throughout the day.

Be creative. There's a delicate balancing act between healthy habits, which by their very nature are routine, and boredom. If walking is your main physical activity, then this might be a time to branch out to cycling. If you're eating the same ten foods for breakfast, lunch, and dinner, check out some magazines or cookbooks for new recipes. Or come to the Lean Plate Club Web chat at www.washingtonpost.com, where members share their recipes each week, and where you can also receive free electronic tools including spreadsheets to help track calories and more. In other words, look for ways to invigorate yourself.

Recruit a buddy. Being accountable to someone else means that it's not so easy to skip a workout. Another option: Consider a session or two with a personal trainer.

Richmond, Va.: I have maintained a slow weight loss of about 50 pounds for a year and a half. Oftentimes, I can't predict how late I will need to stay at work, and I find that keeping individual bags of nuts in my work desk is very helpful. Planters sells some (unsalted) with two servings in them, about 320 calories. I enjoy the bags of walnuts. Eating a bag while I'm working late helps to keep me from pigging out on a late and large dinner when I arrive home.

Mix things up. Cross training helps create muscle "confusion" so that plateaus—and boredom—are less likely to occur. Do the weight machines at the gym in a new order. Walk a different route to work. Work out at a different time of day. Get a pedometer to help boost activities like walking and taking the stairs. You get the idea.

Test yourself. If you've really instilled a healthy new habit, then you can do it no matter what. That means whether you're tired, sad, angry, stressed out, bored, or on vacation. If you can accomplish that, then you can be confident that you can stick with your new habit. Another test is to see if you can overcome the temptation to slip into your old, bad habits with nary a thought. In other words, when you can see the dessert cart and it's not calling your name after a three-course dinner, when you can haul yourself out of bed to work out without thinking about it, when you can eat a small bag of chips and not feel like the large size is gnawing at your soul, then you know that you have turned a short-term change into a long-term habit.

North Bethesda, Md.: I'm a foodaholic when it comes to certain foods. I manage to (mostly) control urges by not keeping those foods around, or if I must have them in the house for my husband, I keep them out of my sight in the basement. My personal strategies are to keep fruit on the counter (two pieces, both of which must be gone before dinner), keep exercising (I now do water fitness twice a week, and the pool will be open even if classes are not in session), and weigh in daily so I can catch any upswing in weight early.

NIGHTTIME EATING

If you nibble at the chocolate cake after dinner and then the meat loaf and then have a spoonful of ice cream and then go back to the cake, and so on, you could be exhibiting some classic signs of nighttime eating syndrome (NES). Do it once or twice and it's no big deal. But if you find that the habit grows—as does your waistline—then it's worth taking a closer look before this pattern undermines all your hard work.

First described in 1955 by University of Pennsylvania psychiatrist Albert Stunkard, NES is an eating disorder that many scientists believe contributes to overweight and obesity.

How many people suffer from the condition is not known. But

estimates are that about 5 percent of those attending obesity clinics have NES, as do up to 28 percent of those awaiting gastric bypass surgery, one of the most drastic treatments for excess weight.

Symptoms can range from occasional nighttime bouts of overeating to nightly binges. At its extreme, the syndrome has these symptoms: skipping breakfast at least four times per week, consuming more than half your daily calories after 7 P.M., and then having difficulty falling asleep or staying asleep more than four nights per week (often because you are so full from eating). Nighttime depression is also very common among NES sufferers.

For years, Stunkard thought NES was caused by disordered sleep. But the latest findings point to a problem with circadian eating rhythms that delays hunger and meals by about six hours. So people with NES are out of sync with the rest of the world. They often don't get hungry for breakfast until late in the morning, which sets off a delayed eating cycle. By nighttime they're ravenous.

A preliminary study found that the antidepressant sertraline (Zoloft) helped treat severe cases of NES. Until experts sort out whether medication really works for NES, here's what they say can help with out-of-control nighttime eating:

Eat breakfast. Most people with NES aren't hungry in the morning. But if you can learn to stomach a morning meal, it can help stop—or at least reduce—nighttime overeating.

Control portions. This is one way to help keep calories in check. If you find yourself succumbing to the urge for evening noshing, have some food. Just measure out portions before eating and stop when that portion is finished.

Keep trigger foods out of the house. The less temptation, the better. You know best what food is likely to call to you at your weakest moment. So load up on low-calorie, filling fare (raw veggies, fruit, soup) that can be consumed if the urge to eat surfaces. And there's no need to avoid favorite foods altogether. Just buy a single serving that can be eaten once or twice a week.

Practice relaxation. A 2003 study by researchers at the Medical University of South Carolina in Charleston found that people with NES who practiced 20 minutes of daily progressive muscle relaxation significantly reduced stress, anxiety, and levels of the stress hormone cortisol in just a week compared with controls. They felt hungrier in the morning, so they were more likely to eat breakfast and start the day well. They engaged in less nighttime eating, and reported less depression and anger than controls.

Find alternatives to eating. Make a list of non-food-related activities to do when the urge for nighttime eating hits. Knit. Call a friend. Work on a photo album. Do a few push-ups or sit-ups. Stretch. Meditate. Exercise while watching television (instead of mindlessly eating). You get the idea.

FOOD CRAVINGS

There's the gooey chocolate chip cookie that calls your name. The bag of salty taco chips that seems irresistible. That unmistakable yearning for a juicy burger and fries, a hot fudge sundae, or a slice of pepperoni pizza.

Food cravings are modern sirens that research shows regularly beckon 97 percent of women and 68 percent of men. Since few of us hanker for asparagus—unless, of course, it's topped with hollandaise sauce—cravings fuel chronic overconsumption of calories and help widen waistlines.

Many who fall under a food's spell often say that they crave it for some unmet nutritional need. To test that theory, researchers at the Monell Chemical Senses Center, a private research facility in Philadelphia, put a group of healthy young adults on a liquid diet that provided plenty of calories and all the essential vitamins and minerals. Despite having all their nutritional needs met, study participants still craved certain foods, suggesting that cravings are not fueled by nutritional deficits.

So as you can see, people don't crave chocolate for its magnesium or porterhouse steak because of the iron it provides. But their bodies are sending a powerful message of psychological desire to the brain. Often craving reflects stress, fatigue, boredom, anger, joy, or a combination of all of the above. The body usually compensates by craving food that is rich in sugar and fat—the reason that you find bowls of candy or nuts, not celery, cherry tomatoes, and baby carrots—strategically placed on office desks. There's good reason for that: Fat and sugar seem to boost the brain's production of endorphins, the so-called feel-good chemicals. Think of food cravings as a form of self-medication.

As you might have anticipated—or experienced firsthand—men and women often feel cravings differently. Men are more likely to desire mixtures of protein, fat, and salt, such as roast beef, hot dogs, pizza, steak, and chips. Women yearn more often for sweet, high-carbohydrate, high-fat foods: cookies, ice cream, pasta, bread. And chocolate is usually in the top five foods that women crave.

Since deadlines aren't likely to disappear and neither is stressful living, here are some ways to help mute the call of food cravings.

Trick, not just treat. People generally crave foods with at least three calories per gram. So when a craving surfaces, try fulfilling it with the lowest-calorie food possible. Think chocolate sorbet instead of chocolate ice cream; salted popcorn or pretzels instead of chips; oven-fried chicken rather than deep-fat fried.

Distract yourself. Time can weaken even the strongest cravings. When a yearning for chocolate chip cookies arises, waiting just 15 to 20 minutes and getting involved in another activity will sometimes allow a craving to pass. Physical activity—walking up and down a few flights of stairs in your building, taking a stroll around the block—can serve as both a distraction and a help to diminish cravings.

Variety really is the spice. In the Monell study of food cravings, participants drank a slightly sweet vanilla-flavored beverage that fulfilled all their daily nutritional needs. The researchers thought this regimen would dull food cravings. But the study found that participants' cravings rose three to four times higher for salty and other nonsweet foods. People often crave something that differs in sensory quality from their normal diet—yet another reason to eat a wide variety of food with different tastes and textures.

Go for the real thing. Instead of trying to eat your way past the craving with other foods, have what you really want. Just make it a small portion. Get the food with the most intense possible taste for your craving, like a chocolate truffle or a small square of bitter chocolate. Sometimes, cravings are simply not satisfied except by the real thing.

Keep tempting foods away when you're feeling susceptible to a food craving. That way, when they beckon, you'll have to go out of your way to get them. Just seeing the food—or getting a whiff of a something you love to eat—can also help trigger cravings and undermine resolve. If you do still indulge in one of your trigger foods, buy a single serving—an ice cream cone, one candy bar, or a small order of fries—that can be consumed in one sitting.

Deconstruct your craving. Most overwhelming desires for food mask other emotional states, for example, feeling tired, stressed, bored, anxious, or angry. Analyze what's going on and then take action. Take a nap if you're really tired, or at least lie down for a few minutes. Take a walk to cope with stress, or simply climb the stairs in your building. And if you're angry, bored, or otherwise at your wit's end, think about calling a friend, your significant other, or a family member simply to talk for a few minutes.

SECRET EXERCISES

Controlling your eating for long-term success is important. But you also need to pay attention to the other side of the weight equation: activity. You've learned in the last eight weeks how to be active for 30 minutes each day. You are now stretching regularly and you lift weights several times a week.

This is a wonderful start. But you'll need to keep branching out to keep your workouts fresh and to keep toning those muscles that have likely been pretty flabby until now. A few simple additional activities can help you preserve posture, protect your back, and maybe even reduce your risk of injuries. These exercises strengthen core muscles—a diverse group that not only supports your trunk but also helps hold your vital organs in place.

Core muscles range from your upper thighs to the pectorals in your chest. They include surface muscles as well as your deep abdominal and back muscles. They're the muscles that are used in just about everything that you do.

While infomercials and gyms hawk a wide variety of equipment and methods to help strengthen core muscles, active everyday living goes a long way toward toning them. "Use them or lose them" really is the trite but true mantra of core muscles. If you live like a couch potato, your core muscles will be slack and able to do only the kinds of sedentary activity that a couch potato does. But if you condition them—even a little—you can see big improvements, since core muscles respond surprisingly quickly to activity. Here are some of ways you can strengthen and tone your core muscles:

Take the stairs. Ditto for walking and other simple lifestyle exercises, like hoofing it to the farthest water fountain or restroom from your desk. Or delivering messages by hand instead of using the phone or e-mail. Being upright, rather than sitting slumped over in a chair, helps tone core muscles. So try to move at least once an hour from your desk.

Do "executive" sit-ups. Here's the perfect activity for the times when you can't leave your chair. Simply pull in your gut. Hold for about 10 to 15 seconds while taking care not to hold your breath. Repeat throughout the day, gradually building up to holding stomach muscles for 60 seconds per rep.

Bird-dog it. In other words, get down on your hands and knees, point your right arm forward, and raise your left leg behind you. Hold while breathing for about 15 seconds. Repeat on the other side. Gradually increase your hold in this position. Push-ups of all kinds also strengthen your core muscles, as do planks. (Lie on your stomach. Raise your body on your forearms and toes, keeping your stomach, buttocks, and other muscles tight so that you don't droop. Hold for about ten seconds—or as long as you can at first—then gradually build up the time.

Look beneath the crunches. Sure, traditional sit-ups, leg raises, and ab crunches will tone, but they won't give you six-pack abs unless you also reach a healthy weight. Extra pounds frequently accumulate around the waist. You may think that it's just your stomach muscles that are weak when it's really the layer of fat that is protruding. Getting to a healthier weight will help reduce that layer of fat.

Reach for the ceiling. Stretching upward helps strengthen some core muscles. When you sit for long periods of time, you tend to shorten core muscles. Just by improving your posture and sitting up straight, you can help keep those core muscles strengthened and elongated.

Easy does it. Whether you lift weights at the gym or perch on an exercise ball at your desk, each activity takes time for your body and brain to learn. The more sedentary you have been, the more your body and brain need to relearn activities. A common mistake is doing too much too soon. You may have been an athlete in your youth, but unless you've stayed active and fit since then, you are likely an athlete only in your mind. Until, that is, you take steps to change that fact.

Fifteen

RECIPES

PUT IT INTO PRACTICE

There's no one menu and no one food that will guarantee you a healthier weight. That's why the Lean Plate Club is grounded in moderation, variety, and choosing plenty of healthy, great-tasting foods that appeal to your particular tastes.

With that in mind, here is a sampler of menus and some recipes for you to use as a starting point. Try them. Tinker with them. Or review them and send your thoughts to my weekly Lean Plate Club Web chat, Tuesdays from 1 to 2 P.M. EST at www.washingtonpost.com, where I give out a handful of prizes each week to participants. You can also share your healthy recipes or healthy food finds or ways to move more with other Lean Plate Club members.

Thinking and acting like a thinner person is an ongoing effort, not something that you do one day, one week, or one month and then return to your old habits. It's a change for life.

You can also e-mail me anytime at leanplateclub@washpost.com. I read all my e-mails and letters and respond personally to as many as time allows.

DO THE NUMBERS

If you can plan a day's worth of meals, you can stay ahead of the numbers game. Here's how to figure it:

1. Take your total number of calories for the day.

2. Divide by the number of meals you plan to eat, which gives you the total per meal.

Calories	1,200	1,400	1,600	1,800	2,000	2,200	2,400
Breakfast	400	466	533	600	666	733	800
Lunch	400	466	533	600	666	733	800
Dinner	400	466	533	600	666	733	800

Few people eat just three meals per day, however. Someone consuming 1,200 calories per day might snack or have other eating preferences similar to those shown below:

	Three square meals	Three meals with snacks	Six small meals	Slow but steady	Dinner lover	Big breakfast eater
Breakfast	400	300	250	200	150	500
Snack	——	100	100	200	150	——
Lunch	400	350	250	200	300	400
Snack	——	100	250	100	——	——
Dinner	400	350	250	400	500	300
Snack		——	100	100	100	——
Total	1,200	1,200	1,200	1,200	1,200	1,200

SAMPLER OF SOURCES FOR HEALTHY MEALS

There are thousands of healthful recipes available free of charge online. Here's a sampling of some good places to find them. Find more each week in the Lean Plate Club Web chat at www.lean plateclub.com.

- **American Institute for Cancer Research**, www.aicr.org. Founded in 1982, this nonprofit organization has grown into the nation's leading charity in the field of diet, nutrition, and cancer. AICR supports research into the role of diet and nutrition in the prevention and treatment of cancer. It offers a wide range of cancer-prevention education programs and provides recipes and nutritional guidance to help consumers reduce their risk of cancer. AICR's latest cookbook is *The New American Cookbook.*

- **5 to 9 a Day program**, www.5aday.gov/recipes/index.html, from the National Cancer Institute encourages consumption of fruits and vegetables. Search online for recipes by ingredient, meal, preparation time, and number of servings of fruits and vegetables per person.

- **The DASH (Dietary Approaches to Stop Hypertension) Eating Plan**, www.nhlbi.nih.gov/health/public/heart/hbp/dash/index.htm, from the National Heart, Lung, and Blood Institute has been proved to help reduce blood pressure as much as some blood-pressure-lowering medication. Find plenty of low-fat, low-cholesterol, low-sodium, and high-potassium recipes.

- **"Delicious Heart Healthy Latino Recipes,"** www.nhlbi.nih.gov/health/public/heart/other/sp_recip.htm, are available in Spanish and English from the National Heart, Lung, and Blood Institute.

- *Heart-Healthy Home Cooking African American Style,* www.nhlbi.nih.gov/health/public/heart/other/chdblack/cooking.htm. This is another publication of the National Heart, Lung, and Blood Institute.

- *Keep the Beat: Heart Healthy Recipes,* www.nhlbi.nih.gov/health/public/heart/other/ktb_recipebk, from the National Heart, Lung, and Blood Institute. To order booklets ($4, 145 pages) by credit card, call the NHLBI Health Information Center, 301-592-8573. Item number 03-2921.

- **Meatless Monday,** www.meatlessmonday.com, is a nonprofit national campaign and Web site developed by the Johns Hopkins School of Public Health in conjunction with twenty-eight other schools of public health, including Columbia University's Mailman School of Public Health. The campaign's goal is to encourage more consumption of fruits, vegetables, and whole grains to help prevent heart disease, stroke, and cancer, and to slowly decrease consumption of meat.

- *Stay Young at Heart,* www.nhlbi.nih.gov/health/public/heart/other/syah/index.htm. This booklet from the National Heart, Lung, and Blood Institute contains 12 recipes. The booklet is available for $0.50, including shipping and handling, by calling 301-592-8573, or by check or money order from the NHLBI Information Center, P.O. Box 30105, Bethesda, MD, 20824-0105. Ask for item number 55-648.

- **Whole Grains Council,** www.wholegrainscouncil.org, is a nonprofit consortium of industry, scientists, chefs, and the nonprofit Oldways Preservation Trust. Based in Boston, the council is committed to increasing consumption of whole grains for better health.

- **World's Healthiest Foods,** www.whfoods.com, is a Web site run by the George Mateljan Foundation. Find healthy recipes, as well as extensive details about their nutritional content, and more about healthful eating.

RECIPE TABLE OF CONTENTS

BREAK THE FAST: BREAKFAST FOOD AND DRINK

No meal seems to be more important to achieving a healthier weight than breakfast. After a night of sleep and fasting, your body needs food. Fuel up well and you set the right tone for the whole day. Make smart choices and you'll not only keep your energy high, but there's good evidence to suggest that you'll also improve your mental performance.

So whether you grab an energy or cereal bar with a glass of milk as you head out the door or you take the time to enjoy a sit-down meal, make sure that you eat breakfast. If your stomach has a hard time waking up, have something very light at home—a half cup of yogurt or half a slice of whole-grain toast—then plan to have a full breakfast in the next couple of hours.

Your morning meal need not be traditional breakfast food. Until the twentieth century, when ready-to-eat cereals were introduced, it was standard practice to eat whatever was left over from the previous night's dinner. So it's perfectly okay to think outside the cereal box. Just try to fuel your body in the morning.

BREAKFAST PIZZA

1 whole wheat pita or whole-grain tortilla
1–2 tablespoons tomato sauce (optional)
¼ cup grated part-skim-milk mozzarella (or nonfat mozzarella)
slices of chicken or turkey sausage or slice of a meat substitute
  sausage

1. Place the pita on a plate. Top with tomato sauce (if desired). Add the cheese. Add the slices of sausage.
2. Microwave on high until the cheese is melted. Serve immediately.

Nutritional info per serving: 300 calories, 8 grams total fat, 4 grams saturated fat, 0 grams trans fats, 18 milligrams cholesterol, 515 milligrams sodium, 36 grams carbohydrates, 5 grams fiber, 1 gram sugars, 15 grams protein.

READY-TO-EAT CEREAL

1 cup whole-grain, unsweetened cereal or very lightly sweetened
  cold cereals (examples: Shredded Wheat, Cheerios, Wheaties,
  Bran Flakes, Wheat Chex, Rice Chex, Corn Chex, Kashi 7
  Whole Grain Flakes, Kashi 7 Whole Grain Pilaf, Kashi 7
  Whole Grain Puffs, Kashi Heart to Heart Cereal)
½–1 cup fresh fruit
1 cup skim or 1 percent milk
2 teaspoons slivered almonds

Nutritional info per serving: Numbers will vary according to what you choose, but this combination provides about 25 percent of the recommended level of calcium and healthy fat (from the almonds), between one to two servings of fruit (a good step toward the 2 cups recommended daily), and a good amount of fiber. Calories range from about 300 to 450.

OATMEAL

1 cup oatmeal (instant, steel cut, quick—it doesn't matter what kind)
skim milk (to boost protein and calcium)
1 tablespoon raisins (or any other dried or fresh fruit) or 1 teaspoon honey or brown sugar

Nutritional info per serving: 230 calories, 3 grams total fat, 1 gram saturated fat, 0 grams trans fats, 5 milligrams cholesterol, 176 milligrams sodium, 37 grams carbohydrates, 4 grams fiber, 18 grams sugars, 12 grams protein.

BAKED OATMEAL

1 cup skim milk
1 teaspoon vanilla extract
¼ cup raisins or other dried fruit of your choice, or mashed banana
½ cup unsweetened applesauce
1 egg, 2 egg whites, or ¼ cup egg substitute
2 cups uncooked quick oats
1½ teaspoons baking powder
¼ teaspoon ground cinnamon
¼ cup dark brown sugar

1. Preheat oven to 350°.

2. Mix wet and dry ingredients separately, then fold in together.

3. Spoon the batter into a nonstick muffin tin (or one lined with paper liners).

4. Bake 35–40 minutes.

Serves 6

Nutritional info per serving: 207 calories, 4 grams total fat, 1 gram saturated fat, 0 grams trans fats, 71 milligrams cholesterol, 46 milligrams sodium, 37 grams carbohydrates, 3 grams fiber, 18 grams sugars, 8 grams protein.

EGGS (OMELET, FRITTATA, SCRAMBLED, POACHED, HARD-BOILED, ETC.)

After spending years out of favor, eggs are cracking open nutritional barriers as a low-cost source of protein. Eggs are also rich in key vitamins and minerals, including iron, and they contain lutein, a substance that appears to help protect vision. Eggs are low in saturated fat and have no trans fats. But a large egg contains 212 milligrams of cholesterol—more than a day's worth for people who have high blood cholesterol levels, heart disease, or diabetes. Because eggs also contain saturated fat and cholesterol, some people need to limit their egg consumption. Even then, there are plenty of other egg-based options, from Egg Beaters to egg whites, now sold in many dairy cases.

Serve your eggs with a slice of whole wheat toast. Scoop them into a whole wheat wrap, or make a "pocket" sandwich with a whole-grain pita or by folding the cooked eggs into a flatbread. The list goes on and on.

WAFFLES, PANCAKES, AND FRENCH TOAST

You can make these from scratch if you have time, but there are a number of healthy options available in the supermarket freezer section. Look for whole-grain varieties that are also low-fat. They can be popped into the toaster or heated in the microwave. Add fresh fruit, a dollop of yogurt, a little maple syrup or honey and serve with a glass of skim milk or low-fat soy milk to add protein to your fast—and, of course, great-tasting—meal.

Other options: Serve with a half cup of unsweetened applesauce, or fruit cup packed in juice, or a half glass of calcium-fortified juice.

BLUEBERRY MUFFIN SQUARES

This high-protein version of a familiar favorite is designed to increase satiety. Courtesy of Holly Edelbrock, Allison Shircliff, and Barbara Burke of the Clinical Research Center at the University of Washington, www.crc.washington.edu. Used by permission.

1 box fat-free Krusteaz Blueberry Muffin mix
1 can blueberries, strained (found inside the muffin mix box)
2½ cups nonfat dry milk
¾ cup Egg Beaters or any egg substitute brand, or ¾ cup egg whites
½ cup + 2 tablespoons safflower oil
¼ cup water

1. Preheat oven to 375°.
2. Combine the mix, blueberries, and nonfat dry milk. Add the eggs, oil, and water, and mix until moistened.
3. Divide the batter into two oiled 9" × 9" pans. Bake 15–18 minutes, or until done. Cool.

Makes 16 squares

Nutritional info per square: 220 calories, 10 grams total fat, 1 gram saturated fat, 0 grams trans fats, 2 milligrams cholesterol, 285 milligrams sodium, 26 grams carbohydrates, 1 gram fiber, 6 grams protein.

APPETIZERS, SOUPS, AND STEWS

Appetizers, soups, and stews offer opportunities to start a meal right. Serve large portions of soups and stews and you've got a one-dish meal. They're filled with multiple flavors that will help satisfy your taste buds, and they can help you feel full and satisfied—a winning combination.

GREEN GAZPACHO SOUP

Mark Miller, chef and owner of the Coyote Café in Sante Fe, New Mexico, has been a trailblazer in presenting Southwestern, Latin/South American, and Asian foods through a string of successful restaurants in the United States, Japan, and Australia. He is the author of several cookbooks, including *The Coyote Café*, and is also a recipient of the James Beard Award for Best Chef–Southwest and numerous other awards.

This gazpacho with a new twist is a recommendation of Countdown USA Recipe, a joint effort of VHA Inc. (formerly the Voluntary Hospitals of America, Inc.) and the James Beard Foundation. It is low in sodium, fat, and cholesterol. Calorie count is approximate because of varying ingredients and serving sizes.

25–30 fresh tomatillos, husked and washed
1 medium red onion
2 cloves garlic

1 *English cucumber, or 2 regular cucumbers*
2 *poblano peppers, roasted, peeled, and seeded*
20 *sprigs cilantro, leaves only*
ice water, if necessary
salt (if desired)
3 *or 4 serrano chilies*
½ *cup nonfat or low-fat plain yogurt*
2 *fresh limes*

1. Save 4 unblemished tomatillos for garnish. Coarsely chop the rest, then place them in a blender or food processor.

2. Chop ¾ of the onion, the garlic, ¾ of the cucumber, the poblanos, and the cilantro. Add to the tomatillos. (If regular cucumbers are used, peel and seed.)

3. Puree. Add ice water to thin if necessary and add salt if desired. Chill.

4. Very finely mince the remaining tomatillos, onion, cucumber, and serrano chilies for salsa garnish. If desired, add salt to taste.

5. Taste the gazpacho. Adjust seasoning and consistency as needed by adding more ice or vegetables.

6. Serve in chilled bowls. Add a dollop of yogurt and a tablespoon or more of the salsa on top of each bowl. Garnish with lime wedges.

Serves 4

Nutritional info per serving: 156 calories, 3 grams total fat, <1 gram saturated fat, 0 grams trans fats, 0 milligrams cholesterol, 25 milligrams sodium, 30 grams carbohydrates, 8 grams fiber, 20 grams sugars, 7 grams protein. It's also an excellent source of vegetables, potassium, lutein, and zeaxanthin, and a good source of vitamin C.

SUGAR SNAP PEA SOUP WITH BASIL AND GARLIC

Named Best Chef–California by the James Beard Foundation, Bradley Ogden has also been named Chef of the Year by the Culinary Institute of America. His restaurant, the Lark Creek Inn in Marin County, north of San Francisco, has been named one of the best restaurants in the country. His latest restaurant—Bradley Ogden at Caesars Palace in Las Vegas—received the James Beard Foundation's Best New Restaurant of the Year award in 2004.

This soup is recommended by Countdown USA Recipe. It is low in sodium, fat, and cholesterol. Calorie count is approximate because of varying ingredients and serving sizes.

Basil and Garlic Puree
½ cup fresh basil leaves
2 cloves garlic, peeled
pinch of kosher salt
1 tablespoon soup cooking liquid
1 teaspoon olive oil
¼ teaspoon fresh ground pepper

Soup
⅔ cup diced carrots
⅔ cup diced leeks, white part only
⅔ cup diced new potato
1½ quarts chicken stock, water, or a combination
1 teaspoon kosher salt
¼ cup broken dried semolina pasta (without eggs)
¼ cup diced red chard stems
½ cup red chard leaves
1 cup diced sugar snap peas (remove all strings before dicing)
fresh ground black pepper

Puree

1. Wash and dry the basil.
2. Mash the garlic with salt until almost pureed.
3. Put the basil, garlic, and remaining puree ingredients in a food processor or blender. Puree until the basil is finely chopped.

Soup

1. Place the carrots, leeks, potato, liquid, and salt in a medium saucepan and bring to a simmer over medium heat.
2. Reduce the heat and cook slowly until the vegetables are almost tender, about 10 minutes.
3. Add the pasta and red chard stems and continue simmering until the pasta is just cooked, 5–10 minutes.
4. Just before serving add the chard leaves and diced peas.
5. Simmer 3–4 minutes, or until the peas are cooked al dente.
6. Ladle into soup bowls and top each serving with ½ teaspoon of the basil and garlic puree and pepper.

Serves 6

Nutritional info per serving: 80 calories, 2.5 grams total fat, <1 gram saturated fat, 0 grams trans fats, 0 milligrams cholesterol, 576 milligrams sodium (less with low-sodium broth or water), 10 grams carbohydrates, 2 grams fiber, 1.5 grams sugars, 5 grams protein.

BRAZILIAN-STYLE SEAFOOD STEW

From *The New American Cookbook: Recipes for a Healthy Weight and a Healthy Life* by the American Institute for Cancer Research. Used by permission.

¾ *pound skinless white fish fillets (such as halibut, cod, or red snapper) cut into 1" pieces*
salt and freshly ground white pepper
3 tablespoons olive oil, divided

2 tablespoons freshly squeezed lime juice

3 garlic cloves, finely minced

1½ cups chopped onion

½ cup chopped green bell pepper

½ cup chopped red bell pepper

½ cup chopped orange bell pepper

1 fresh serrano chili, seeded and diced (wear rubber gloves to handle fresh chilies, and keep your hands away from your eyes), or ¾ teaspoon cayenne, to taste

1 garlic clove, mashed

1 can (14½ ounces) diced tomatoes in juice

¾ cup unsweetened, reduced-fat coconut milk

½ cup finely chopped fresh cilantro, loosely packed, divided

½ cup finely chopped fresh chives, loosely packed, divided

¾ pound medium shrimp, peeled and deveined

3 cups hot cooked long-grain brown rice

1. Sprinkle the fish with salt and pepper and let it stand a few minutes.

2. In a large bowl, whisk together 2 tablespoons of the olive oil and the lime juice. Stir in the minced garlic. Add the fish and stir to coat on all sides. Let stand for 15 minutes.

3. In a large pot, heat the remaining 1 tablespoon of oil over medium heat. Add the onion, bell peppers, chili, and mashed garlic. Sauté for about 5 minutes, stirring often, until the onion is translucent.

4. Mix in the tomatoes with juice, coconut milk, ¼ cup of the cilantro, ¼ cup of the chives, shrimp, and the fish and its marinade. Bring the liquid to a simmer and cook gently for 5–7 minutes, until the fish and shrimp are opaque in the center. Take care not to overcook the seafood. Season to taste with salt and pepper.

5. Place ½ cup of hot cooked rice in each of 6 shallow bowls. Ladle the stew on top of the rice. Sprinkle with the remaining cilantro and chives.

Serves 6

Nutritional info per serving: 319 calories, 10 grams total fat, 2 grams saturated fat, 0 grams trans fats, 0 milligrams cholesterol, 220 milligrams sodium, 33 grams carbohydrates, 2 grams fiber, 24 grams protein.

CORN CHOWDER
Adapted from *Keep the Beat: Heart Healthy Recipes,* by the National Heart, Lung, and Blood Institute.

1 tablespoon vegetable oil
2 tablespoons celery, finely diced
2 tablespoons onion, finely diced
2 tablespoons sweet red, yellow, or orange pepper, finely diced
1 package (10 ounces) frozen whole-kernel corn (no sauce added)
1 cup peeled raw potatoes, diced in ½" pieces
1 cup water or low-sodium chicken or vegetable broth
¼ teaspoon salt
ground pepper, to taste
¼ teaspoon paprika
2 cups skim or low-fat milk
2 tablespoons flour or cornstarch
2 tablespoons fresh parsley or cilantro, finely chopped

1. Heat the oil in a medium saucepan. Add the celery, onion, and pepper. Sauté for 2 minutes.
2. Add the corn, potatoes, water or broth, salt, pepper, and

paprika. Bring to a boil, then reduce heat to medium. Cook covered for about 10 minutes, or until potatoes are tender.

3. Place ½ cup of the milk in a jar with a tight-fitting lid. Add the flour or cornstarch and shake vigorously.

4. Gradually add the milk-flour mixture to the cooked vegetables, stirring or using a whisk to blend. Then add the remaining milk.

5. Cook, stirring constantly, until the mixture barely comes to a boil and thickens. Be careful not to scald the milk or burn the bottom of the pot. Serve garnished with fresh parsley or cilantro.

Serves 4 (one cup each)

Nutritional info per serving: 186 calories, 5 grams total fat, 1 gram saturated fat, 0 grams trans fats, 5 milligrams cholesterol, 205 milligrams sodium, 455 milligrams potassium, 31 grams carbohydrates, 4 grams fiber, 7 grams protein.

DRESSINGS

LEAN PLATE CLUB "GREEN GODDESS" DRESSING

Avocados are rich in vitamin E and healthy fat. While this recipe isn't low in calories, it's rich in flavor and healthy ingredients. Plus, the fat in the dressing helps you absorb some of the essential vitamins and phytonutrients in the salad.

2 tablespoons guacamole or 2 tablespoons ripe mashed avocado
2 tablespoons vinegar (balsamic, white balsamic, orange muscat champagne, or raspberry)

Place the guacamole or avocado in a small bowl. Drizzle in the vinegar while whisking.

Serves 2

Nutritional info per serving (approximate): 50 calories, 4 grams total fat, 1 gram saturated fat, 0 grams trans fats, 0 milligrams cholesterol, 44 milligrams sodium, 2 grams carbohydrates, 1 gram fiber, 1 gram protein.

YOGURT SALAD DRESSING

This dressing can be used on lettuce salads, pasta, or whole-grain salads. Adapted from *Keep the Beat: Heart Healthy Recipes*, by the National Heart, Lung, and Blood Institute.

8 ounces fat-free plain yogurt, preferably Greek variety, such as
    Total by Fage, which is very rich and creamy
¼ cup fat-free or low-fat mayonnaise
2 tablespoons dried chives
2 tablespoons dill or cilantro, diced
2 tablespoons lemon juice
salt (as desired)
pepper (as desired), white or black, freshly ground

1. In a bowl, mix all the ingredients together until thoroughly combined.

2. Refrigerate for 1–2 hours to allow the taste of the herbs to "blossom."

Serves 8 (2 tablespoons each)

Nutritional info per serving (using nonfat ingredients): 23 calories, 0 grams total fat, 0 grams saturated fat, 0 grams trans fats, 1 milligram cholesterol, 84 milligrams sodium, 104 milligrams potassium, 4 grams carbohydrates, 0 grams fiber, 2 grams protein.

VINAIGRETTE SALAD DRESSING

Adapted from *Keep the Beat: Heart Healthy Recipes*, by the National Heart, Lung, and Blood Institute.

1 bulb garlic, separated into cloves, peeled
½ cup water
1 tablespoon red wine vinegar
¼ teaspoon honey
1 tablespoon virgin olive oil (or other healthy oil)
½ teaspoon black pepper
salt (to taste)

1. Place the garlic in a small saucepan and pour in enough water to cover the cloves, about ½ cup.

2. Bring the water to a boil. Reduce heat and simmer until the garlic is tender, about 15 minutes.

3. Continue to cook until the liquid is reduced to 2 tablespoons and increase the heat for about 3 minutes.

4. Pour the contents into a small sieve over a bowl. With a wooden spoon, mash the garlic through the sieve (or use a garlic press).

5. Whisk the vinegar into the garlic mixture. Mix in the honey, oil, and seasonings.

Serves 4 (2 tablespoons each)

Nutritional info per serving: 33 calories, 3 grams total fat, 1 gram saturated fat, 0 grams trans fats, 0 milligrams cholesterol, 0 milligrams sodium, 9 milligrams potassium, 1 gram carbohydrates, 0 grams protein, 0 grams fiber.

HOT 'N' SPICY SEASONING

According to the latest government food surveys, nearly everyone eats too much sodium. So even if you don't have high blood pressure, it's a good idea to reduce sodium intake. This seasoning, which can be made in large quantities, keeps best in an airtight container. You can also put it in a shaker to be used in place of— or in addition to—your tabletop saltshakers. Adapted from *Keep the Beat: Heart Healthy Recipes* by the National Heart, Lung, and Blood Institute.

> 1½ teaspoons white pepper
> ½ teaspoon cayenne pepper
> ½ teaspoon black pepper
> 1 teaspoon onion powder
> 1¼ teaspoons garlic powder
> 1 tablespoon dried basil
> 1½ teaspoons dried thyme

Place all the ingredients in a lidded jar. Shake to combine.

Makes ⅓ cup

Nutritional info per serving: 1 calorie, 1 gram total fat, 0 grams saturated fat, 0 grams trans fats, 0 milligrams cholesterol, 0 milligrams sodium, 4 milligrams potassium, <1 gram carbohydrates, 0 grams fiber, 0 grams protein.

SALADS

A well-made salad goes far beyond iceberg lettuce, a pale tomato, and bottled dressing. It can easily offer a day's worth of vegetables and maybe even some fruit. Here are just a few possibilities.

LEAN PLATE CLUB SALAD

1–2 cups mixed greens
½–1 cup cherry or grape tomatoes
3–4 olives, diced
1 tablespoon pickled jalapeño pepper slices
1 sweet pepper, sliced (red, yellow, or orange, or a
     combination)
½ cup cooked or canned beans (kidney, black, red, pinto, or white
     beans), drained
1 ounce low-fat or fat-free feta, goat, or other reduced-fat cheese
     (if you prefer higher fat, use only ½ ounce), crumbled or
     grated
2 celery sticks, diced (or fennel, shaved or diced)
½ cup fruit (strawberries, raspberries, diced apples, sliced pears,
     peaches, mangoes, grapes, papaya)
2 teaspoons slivered almonds (or other nuts)
½ small jar marinated artichoke hearts
⅛–¼ avocado, sliced
1–2 ounces diced lean meat (chicken or turkey without the skin or
     seafood, optional)
2 hard-boiled egg whites, sliced
fresh cilantro, chopped
1 hard-boiled egg yolk (optional)

1. Wash and dry greens.
2. Add other ingredients. Toss.
3. Use dressing of your choice.

Serves 1–2, depending on ingredients

Nutritional info per serving: Calories vary from about 200 to 400 depending on serving and ingredients.

BEAN, CORN, AND PEPPER SALAD WITH CHICKEN

From *The New American Cookbook: Recipes for a Healthy Weight and a Healthy Life* by the American Institute for Cancer Research. Used by permission.

> 1½ cups brown rice (if you're short on time, use quick-cooking brown rice or look in the freezer section of grocery stores for cooked brown rice that requires only about 2 minutes in the microwave to thaw)
>
> 3 cups cubed cooked skinless chicken breast
>
> 1 can (15 ounces) corn, drained (look for reduced sodium or no added sodium)
>
> 1 can (15½ ounces) black beans, rinsed and drained
>
> 1 medium green bell pepper, seeded and diced
>
> 1 medium red bell pepper, seeded and diced
>
> ½ cup peeled and diced jicama
>
> ⅓ cup extra-virgin olive oil
>
> 1 tablespoon freshly squeezed lime juice, or to taste
>
> ¾ cup chunky salsa
>
> 3 drops hot pepper sauce, such as Tabasco, or to taste (optional)
>
> 2–4 tablespoons water
>
> salt and freshly ground black pepper
>
> green leafy lettuce
>
> ¼ cup finely chopped fresh cilantro or flat-leaf parsley, loosely packed, for garnish
>
> ¼ cup low-fat or nonfat shredded Cheddar cheese, for garnish

1. In a large bowl, combine the rice, chicken, corn, beans, bell peppers, and jicama. Gently toss until well mixed. Set aside.

2. In a medium bowl, whisk together the olive oil and lime juice until well blended. Mix in the salsa and hot pepper sauce. Add enough water to thin the consistency so the dressing can be thinly drizzled over the salad. Drizzle the dressing over the

chicken mixture and toss to coat the salad ingredients evenly. Cover the salad and refrigerate for 1–3 hours so the flavors can meld.

3. Bring the salad to room temperature and check the seasonings before serving. Season to taste with salt and pepper. Drain off any excess dressing. Place the salad in a serving bowl lined with lettuce leaves. Sprinkle with cilantro or parsley and cheese.

Serves 6

Nutritional info per serving: 395 calories (slightly fewer if you use nonfat Cheddar), 15 grams total fat, 2 grams saturated fat, 0 grams trans fats, 691 milligrams sodium, 40 grams carbohydrates, 7 grams fiber, 29 grams protein.

COUSCOUS SALAD

This high-protein version of a familiar favorite is designed to help increase satiety. Courtesy of Holly Edelbrock, Allison Shircliff, and Barbara Burke of the Clinical Research Center at the University of Washington, www.crc.washington.edu. Used by permission.

1 teaspoon onion powder
2 teaspoons fresh garlic, minced
2 teaspoons chicken bouillon granules
1½ tablespoons olive oil
1 cup dry couscous
1½ cups water
1½ tablespoons lemon juice
2 cups fresh or frozen peppers
1 pound cooked chicken breast

1. Combine the spices, bouillon granules, oil, and couscous in a medium bowl.

2. Put the water in a microwavable container and microwave until boiling (about 2–3 minutes). Add the boiling water and lemon juice to the couscous mixture.

3. Cover with plastic wrap and let sit for 5 minutes; fluff with a fork.

4. Add the peppers and chicken to the couscous and stir. Serve hot or cold.

Serves 4

Nutritional information per serving: 360 calories, 8 grams total fat, 2 grams saturated fat, 0 grams trans fats, 84 milligrams cholesterol, 551 milligrams sodium, 33 grams carbohydrates, 3 grams fiber, 36 grams protein.

BASIC BULGUR
Used by permission of the Whole Grains Council and Oldways Preservation Trust.

2 cups broth or water
1 cup bulgur

1. In a saucepan, bring the broth or water to a boil.

2. Add the bulgur and simmer, covered, for about 12 minutes, or until all the liquid is absorbed. Fluff with a fork.

Serves 4

Nutritional info per serving: 57 calories, <1 gram total fat, 0 grams saturated fat, 0 grams trans fats, 0 milligrams cholesterol, 38 milligrams sodium (if made with low-sodium broth), 10 grams carbohydrates, 2 grams fiber, 0 grams sugars, 4 grams protein.

BULGUR–BLACK BEAN SALAD

Used by permission of Cynthia Harriman, the Whole Grains Council and Oldways Preservation Trust.

  1 cup uncooked bulgur
  2 cups water or broth
  1 orange
  2 teaspoons vinegar
  2 tablespoons canola or olive oil
  ½ teaspoon ground cumin
  1 can (14–15 ounces) black beans, rinsed and drained
  1 red bell pepper, chopped in small pieces
  6 stalks green onions, chopped
  4 tablespoons fresh parsley, chopped

1. Put the bulgur and water or broth in a covered saucepan. Bring to a boil, then simmer 10–12 minutes, or until all the liquid is absorbed. Let the bulgur cool, then fluff with a fork.

2. Scrub the orange, then grate the top colored layer of rind (a cheese grater works fine if you don't have a citrus zester).

3. Cut the orange in half and squeeze the juice into a large mixing bowl.

4. Add the orange rind, vinegar, oil, and cumin to the orange juice.

5. Add the beans and veggies to the bowl and mix. Add the cooked bulgur and mix again to combine everything.

6. Chill in the refrigerator a half hour or more before serving.

Serves 4

Variations
• Use leftover cooked bulgur from last night's dinner.
• Substitute whole wheat couscous for the bulgur.

- Try different vegetables—be creative.
- Use a lemon instead of an orange.

Nutritional info per serving: 285 calories, 8 grams total fat, 1 gram saturated fat, 0 grams trans fats, 0 milligrams cholesterol, 459 milligrams sodium (if made with low-sodium broth), 44 grams carbohydrates, 14 grams fiber, 5 grams sugars, 13 grams protein.

MAIN COURSES

Slimmed-down versions of favorite foods can help you control your calories and still savor meals. Here is a taste of some of the healthy recipes available for main courses.

BARBECUED CHICKEN SPICY SOUTHERN STYLE
Adapted from *Keep the Beat: Heart Healthy Recipes*, by the National Heart, Lung, and Blood Institute.

5 tablespoons (3 ounces) tomato paste
1 teaspoon ketchup
2 teaspoons honey
1 teaspoon molasses
1 teaspoon Worcestershire sauce
4 teaspoons white vinegar
¾ teaspoon cayenne pepper
⅛ teaspoon freshly ground black pepper
¼ teaspoon onion powder
2 cloves garlic, minced
⅛ teaspoon grated ginger root
1½ pounds boneless, skinless chicken thighs and breasts

1. In a small pan over medium-low heat combine all the ingredients except the chicken. Cook for 15 minutes. Remove from the heat and let cool.

2. Wash the chicken pieces and pat dry with paper towels. Place the chicken on a large platter and coat evenly with half the sauce. Cover with plastic wrap and refrigerate for 1 hour.

3. Preheat the broiler. Line a broiler pan with foil and place the chicken on the pan. Broil 4–5 minutes on each side.

4. Reduce the oven heat to 350° and spoon the remaining sauce over the chicken. Bake covered for 10 minutes. Remove the thighs and bake the breasts 10 more minutes. Serve hot or cold.

Serves 6 (½ breast or 2 small drumsticks per serving)

Nutritional info per serving: 176 calories, 4 grams total fat, 1 gram saturated fat, 0 grams trans fats, 81 milligrams cholesterol, 199 milligrams sodium, 7 grams carbohydrates, 1 gram fiber, 27 grams protein, 392 milligrams potassium.

BAKED SALMON DIJON

Adapted from *Keep the Beat: Heart Healthy Recipes,* by the National Heart, Lung, and Blood Institute.

Salmon is an excellent source of healthy omega-3 fatty acids and potassium. The mustard in this recipe gives it a nice kick.

1 cup fat-free sour cream
2 teaspoons dried dill (or about 2 tablespoons fresh dill, chopped)
3 tablespoons scallions, finely chopped (both white and green)
2 tablespoons Dijon mustard
2 tablespoons lemon juice
cooking oil spray (as needed)
1½ pounds salmon fillet with skin (fresh or frozen)
½ teaspoon garlic powder
½ teaspoon black pepper
salt to taste

1. Whisk together the sour cream, dill, scallions, mustard, and lemon juice in a small bowl.

2. Preheat the oven to 400°. Lightly oil a nonstick baking sheet with cooking spray.

3. Place the salmon skin-side down on the baking sheet. Sprinkle with garlic powder and pepper, then cover with the sauce.

4. Bake the salmon until just opaque in the center, about 20 minutes. Be sure not to overcook.

Serves 6

Nutritional info per 4-ounce serving: 196 calories, 7 grams total fat, 2 grams saturated fat, 0 grams trans fats, 76 milligrams cholesterol, 229 milligrams sodium, 703 milligrams potassium, <1 gram fiber, 5 grams carbohydrates, 27 grams protein.

SPINACH-STUFFED SOLE

Adapted from *Keep the Beat: Heart Healthy Recipes*, by the National Heart, Lung, and Blood Institute.

cooking oil spray (as needed)
1 teaspoon olive oil
½ pound fresh mushrooms, sliced
½ pound fresh spinach, chopped
¼ teaspoon dried oregano
1 clove garlic, minced
4 six-ounce sole fillets or other white fish
2 tablespoons sherry
4 ounces (1 cup) part-skim-milk mozzarella, grated

1. Preheat the oven to 400°.
2. Coat a 10" × 6" baking dish with the cooking spray.

3. Heat the olive oil in a skillet and sauté the mushrooms for about 3 minutes, or until tender.

4. Add the spinach and continue cooking for about 1 minute, or until the spinach is barely wilted. Remove from heat and drain the liquid into the prepared baking dish.

5. Add the oregano and garlic to the drained, sautéed vegetables. Stir.

6. Divide the vegetable mixture evenly among the fish fillets and place in the center of each. Roll each fillet around the mixture and place seam-side down in the prepared baking dish. Sprinkle with sherry, then place mozzarella grated on top.

7. Bake until the fish flakes easily, about 15–20 minutes.

Serves 4

Nutritional info per serving: 273 calories, 9 grams total fat, 4 grams saturated fat, 0 grams trans fats, 95 milligrams cholesterol, 163 milligrams sodium, 880 milligrams potassium, 6 grams carbohydrates, 2 grams fiber, 39 grams protein.

LASAGNA

This high-protein version of a familiar favorite is designed to help increase satiety. Courtesy of Holly Edelbrock, Allison Shircliff, and Barbara Burke of the Clinical Research Center at the University of Washington, www.crc.washington.edu. Used by permission.

1 pound leanest ground beef (9–10 percent fat)
4 teaspoons dehydrated onion flakes
2 teaspoons fresh garlic, minced
1⅓ cups low-fat marinara sauce
¾ cup tomato paste
8 lasagna noodles

cooking oil spray (as needed)
1½ cups fat-free cottage cheese
12 ounces (3 cups) grated low-fat mozzarella

1. Preheat the oven to 350°.
2. In a medium or large saucepan, brown the ground beef until cooked thoroughly. Add the onion flakes, garlic, marinara sauce, and tomato paste. Mix well. Stir and simmer for 10–15 minutes on low heat.
3. Cook the lasagna noodles according to package directions. Drain well.
4. Spread the sauce in the bottom of an oiled (spray with Pam or other healthy oil spray) 9" × 9" baking pan and layer noodles, sauce, and cottage cheese, finishing with the grated mozzarella. Bake for 30–45 minutes.

Serves 6

Nutritional info per serving: 500 calories, 15 grams total fat, 7 grams saturated fat, 0 grams trans fats, 75 milligrams cholesterol, 730 milligrams sodium, 45 grams carbohydrates, 3 grams fiber, 50 grams protein.

CHICKEN CASSEROLE

Lean chicken breasts and low-fat cheese turn this simple casserole into high-protein fare. Courtesy of Holly Edelbrock, Allison Shircliff, and Barbara Burke of the Clinical Research Center at the University of Washington, www.crc.washington.edu. Used by permission.

4 teaspoons onion flakes
1 teaspoon black pepper
2 teaspoons fresh garlic, minced
1 cup Campbell's Healthy Request Cream of Chicken Soup
2 cups cooked long-grain brown rice

4 cups skinless, boneless chicken breast, cooked and cut into small
   pieces
1 cup frozen artichoke hearts
vegetable spray (as needed)
6½ ounces grated, reduced-fat Cheddar cheese

1. Preheat the oven to 350°.
2. Mix the spices and soup in a large bowl. Add the cooked
rice, chicken, and artichoke hearts and mix thoroughly.
3. Place the mixture in a baking dish sprayed with vegetable
spray. Top with the grated cheese. Bake 30–35 minutes, or until
hot and bubbling.

Serves 4

Nutritional info per serving: 549 calories, 17 grams total fat, 8 grams
saturated fat, 0 grams trans fats, 156 milligrams cholesterol, 756
milligrams sodium, 35 grams carbohydrates, 4 grams fiber, 59 grams
protein.

TUNA CARPACCIO WITH CILANTRO AND GINGER YOGURT

Jeremiah Tower, formerly of Stars Restaurant in San Francisco and
author of *America's Best Chefs Cook with Jeremiah Tower,* developed
this variation of a classic for Countdown USA Recipe, a joint effort
of the Voluntary Hospitals of America, Inc. (now called VHA Inc.)
and the James Beard Foundation. It will give your culinary skills a
mild workout, but is designed to be low in sodium, fat, and cholesterol. Calorie count is approximate because of varying ingredients and serving sizes.

1 tablespoon fresh ginger, finely chopped
6 ounces (¾ cup) low-fat or nonfat plain yogurt

6 *two-ounce paper-thin slices fresh tuna, about 1/16" thick (slice*
thinly or place tuna between two pieces of waxed paper and
tap lightly until thin)
2 *tablespoons fresh lemon juice*
1 *tablespoon fresh cilantro, chopped*
salt (optional)
freshly ground pepper
1/4 *cup olive oil*
12 *cilantro sprigs for garnish*

1. Mix together the ginger and yogurt.

2. Place the tuna on a cold plate and refrigerate to keep cold while preparing the vinaigrette.

3. Combine the lemon juice, chopped cilantro, salt, and pepper in a small bowl. Whisk in the olive oil. Just before serving, pour the vinaigrette over the tuna.

4. Drizzle with the ginger yogurt and garnish with cilantro sprigs

Serves 6

Nutritional info per serving: 130 calories, 10 grams total fat, 1.5 grams saturated fat (with nonfat yogurt), 0 grams trans fats, 13 milligrams cholesterol, 33 milligrams sodium, 2 grams carbohydrates, 0 grams fiber, 8 grams protein.

GRILLED LEG OF LAMB

Award-winning chef Michael Foley, the proprietor and chef at the acclaimed Chicago restaurant Printer's Row for 25 years and author of the upcoming book *Printer's Row: The Evolution of an American Cook,* created this elegant entrée. This recipe is also part of Countdown USA Recipe, a joint effort of the Voluntary Hospitals of America, Inc., (now called VHA Inc.) and the James Beard Foundation.

1 bunch rosemary (reserve 1 sprig for garnish)
2 cloves garlic
2 tablespoons + 1–2 teaspoons extra-virgin olive oil
12 asparagus spears
1 zucchini, cut into strips
1 Japanese eggplant, cut into strips
1 summer (yellow) squash, cut into strips
3 tomatoes, peeled, halved, and seeded
1 head radicchio, quartered
6 shiitake mushrooms
6 scallions
3 pounds boneless leg of lamb

1. Steep the rosemary and garlic in 2 tablespoons of olive oil.
2. Grill or broil all the vegetables. Arrange them on one side of an ovenproof platter.
3. Cut the lamb into 3½-ounce medallions. Brush with the herbed oil. Grill or broil to medium rare.
4. Place the lamb on the platter with the vegetables and place under the broiler briefly, about 30 seconds to 1 minute.
5. Drizzle the lamb with 1–2 teaspoons olive oil and sprinkle with fresh rosemary.

Serves 6

Nutritional info per serving: 410 calories, 18 grams total fat, 6 grams saturated fat, 0 grams trans fats, 142 milligrams cholesterol, 194 milligrams sodium, 11 grams carbohydrates, 4 grams fiber, 5 grams sugars, 49 grams protein.

TANDOORI-STYLE ROAST CHICKEN

For 12 years, cookbook author Joyce Goldstein was the chef/owner of Square One, a well-known Mediterranean restaurant in San

Francisco. She is the author of several cookbooks, including *Italian Slow and Savory, Solo Suppers, Enoteca,* and *Back to Square One: Old World Food in a New World Kitchen,* which earned both the James Beard and Julia Child Awards for Best General Cookbook. With this recipe, no one in your family will complain, "Not chicken *again.*" Serve with saffron rice.

1 onion, cut in chunks
2 cloves garlic, chopped
½ cup lime or lemon juice
1 tablespoon ground coriander
½ teaspoon cayenne pepper
2 teaspoons paprika
1 teaspoon ground ginger
½ teaspoon ground cloves
¼ teaspoon cardamom
½ teaspoon turmeric
½ teaspoon salt
freshly ground black pepper to taste
2 cups plain nonfat or low-fat yogurt
6 baby or spring chickens (poussin) or 6 Cornish hens, each about
    1 pound, or 12 boneless chicken breast halves
1 lime, cut into wedges

1. Puree the onion and garlic in a food processor. Add the lime juice, spices, and yogurt. Process well.

2. Place the chicken in the yogurt mixture and marinate in the refrigerator overnight. (If you're short on time, marinate for several hours.)

3. Remove the chicken from the refrigerator and bring to room temperature.

4. Preheat the oven to 450°. Roast the chicken for 40–45 minutes (or broil or grill).

5. Sprinkle with additional paprika.
6. Garnish with lime wedges.

Serves 12

Nutritional info per serving: 360 calories, 24 grams total fat*, 7 grams saturated fat, 0 grams trans fats; 169 milligrams cholesterol, 113 milligrams sodium, 3 grams carbohydrates, 0 grams fiber, 3 grams sugars, 31 grams protein.

*Cornish hens with skin. To reduce fat, serve hens without skin.

OVEN-ROASTED RED SNAPPER FILLETS WITH TOMATOES AND ONION

He's known simply as Emeril—a name synonymous with fine food and fun cooking. Emeril Lagasse launched his career as the chef at the famed Commander's Palace in New Orleans and now heads a corporation of Emeril restaurants, hosts a television show on the Food Network, and is the author of numerous cookbooks. Recipe courtesy of Emeril Lagasse.

4 four- to six-ounce skin-on red snapper fillets
1 teaspoon salt, plus more to taste
½ teaspoon freshly ground black pepper, plus more to taste
20 (¼" thick) slices Roma tomatoes
¼ cup chiffonade of fresh basil, plus more for garnish, if desired
½ cup julienned sweet onions
¼ cup pitted and sliced Kalamata olives
12 thin slices lemon, seeds removed
2 tablespoons good-quality extra-virgin olive oil

1. Preheat the oven to 400°F and line a baking sheet with parchment paper.

2. Season both sides of the fillets with 1 teaspoon salt and ½ teaspoon pepper. Set aside. Season both sides of the tomato slices with salt and pepper to taste.

3. Arrange 4 rows of 5 tomato slices on the baking sheet so that the tomatoes on each row overlap one another slightly. Sprinkle 1 tablespoon of basil over each row of tomatoes. Distribute the onions and olives evenly over the basil. Place 1 fillet over each group of tomatoes, skin side up. Lay three lemon slices over the top of each fillet. Drizzle 1½ teaspoons of olive oil over each fillet.

4. Bake for 12 to 15 minutes, or until the snapper is cooked through. Serve fillets over rice pilaf (see page 307), distributing the tomatoes, onion, and lemons as well. Garnish each fillet with some chiffonade of fresh basil.

Serves 4

Nutritional info per serving: 275 calories, 12 grams total fat, 2 grams saturated fat, 0 grams trans fats, 63 milligrams cholesterol, 382 milligrams sodium, 4 grams carbohydrates, 1.5 grams fiber, 36 grams protein.

GRILLED HALIBUT WITH STEWED FRESH TOMATOES

Larry Forgione, known as the "godfather of American cuisine," is the founder and chef of An American Place restaurant, now in its fifth incarnation at Lord & Taylor, in New York City. Forgione has earned many awards, including a James Beard Chef of the Year and an Ivy Award (best chef chosen by his peers). This is a Countdown USA Recipe.

4 six- to eight-ounce halibut fillets, skinned
salt to taste
freshly ground black pepper

5 tablespoons olive oil
¼ cup red onion, finely chopped
½ teaspoon garlic, finely chopped
2 cups ripe tomatoes, peeled, seeded, and chopped
¼ cup dry white wine
4 tablespoons parsley, chopped
4 tablespoons basil, chopped

1. Fire up the grill or preheat the broiler.
2. Season each fillet with salt, if desired, and pepper. Brush with 2 tablespoons of the olive oil.
3. In a small saucepan, heat 3 tablespoons of olive oil. Sauté the onion and garlic for 1 minute, taking care not to brown the onion.
4. Stir in the tomatoes and wine. Simmer for 2–3 minutes.
5. Add the parsley and basil. Season with salt and pepper to taste. Set aside, keeping the mixture warm.
6. Grill or broil the fish for 3–4 minutes on each side.
7. Place each fillet in the center of a plate. Spoon the stewed tomato mixture over the halibut.

Serves 4

Nutritional info per serving: 425 calories (7-ounce fillets), 22 grams total fat, 3 grams saturated fat, 0 grams trans fats, 63 milligrams cholesterol, 159 milligrams sodium, 7 grams carbohydrates, 2 grams fiber, 1 gram sugars, 43 grams protein. Good source of lean protein, healthy omega-3 fatty acids, and vitamin C.

GRILLED CHICKEN WITH JAPANESE PEAR APPLES

This unusual chicken dish was created by Madeleine Kamman, a retired award-winning chef and teacher of culinary arts, cofounder with Beringer Vineyards of the School for American Chefs, and author of numerous cookbooks, including *Dinner Against the Clock* and *The Making of a Cook*, which offer a number of healthy and easily prepared dishes. This is a Countdown USA Recipe.

> 6 chicken cutlets (boneless side of the breast)
> 2 tablespoons light soy sauce
> coarsely ground black pepper
> 2 large Japanese pear apples,* washed, cored, and sliced
> 1 tablespoon canola, olive, or safflower oil
> salt (if desired) to taste
> 3 tablespoons slivered scallions

1. Brush the chicken cutlets with soy sauce and pepper them lightly. Let stand 1 hour at room temperature, covered with an upside-down salad strainer to keep flying insects away.

2. Sauté the pear apple slices in oil until nice and brown on each side. Season with salt (if desired) and freshly ground pepper. Remove to a plate to keep warm.

3. Grill or broil the chicken cutlets 2–3 minutes on each side.

4. Slice the chicken cutlets. Alternate slices of chicken with slices of Japanese pear apple.

5. Serve sprinkled with slivered scallions

Serves 6

Nutritional info: 170 calories, 4 grams total fat, <1 gram saturated fat, 0 grams trans fats, 69 milligrams cholesterol, 276 milligrams

---

*Japanese or Chinese pears have a brown skin and a wine-flavored overtone. They are crunchy, like an apple, but as juicy as a just-ripe pear. Find them in Asian groceries, specialty produce markets, and some chain grocery stores. Any other crisp pear or apple that can be sautéed without falling apart during cooking can be used instead of the Oriental fruit. Keeping the skin of the fruit on provides better vitamin intake.

sodium, <1 gram carbohydrates, 1 gram fiber, 3 grams sugars, 27 grams protein.

PORK TENDERLOIN WITH APPLES AND ONION

Jacques Pépin is one of the world's renowned chefs. In addition to his numerous cookbooks, he cohosted a PBS television cooking series with Julia Child and hosted several of his own cooking series. This recipe is from *Simple and Healthy Cooking* and is a Countdown USA Recipe.

4 four-ounce pieces pork tenderloin, completely trimmed of fat, butterflied, and pounded to a thickness of ½"
¾ teaspoon freshly ground black pepper
¼ teaspoon crushed dry thyme
1 tablespoon corn, safflower, or sunflower oil
6 ounces onion, thinly sliced (2 cups)
¼ cup cider vinegar
¼ cup water
1 teaspoon sugar
½ teaspoon ground cumin or caraway seeds
1 pound apples, cored, halved, and thinly sliced (Rome Beauty, if possible)
½ teaspoon salt (if desired)

1. Season the pieces of pork on both sides with ½ teaspoon of pepper and the thyme.
2. Heat the oil in a nonstick skillet over high heat until very hot.
3. Add the pork to the pan and cook 2–3 minutes on each side.
4. Remove the meat from the pan and keep it warm.
5. Add the onion to the pan and sauté for about 3 minutes, until it is softened.
6. In a bowl, mix together the vinegar, water, sugar, and cumin or caraway seeds.

7. Add the vinegar mixture to the pan, along with the apples, salt (if desired), and remaining ¼ teaspoon pepper.

8. Cover and boil gently 4–5 minutes, until the liquid has almost evaporated and the apples are moist and tender.

9. Return the pork and any accumulated juices to the pan and reheat for 1–2 minutes.

Serves 4

Nutritional info per serving: 260 calories, 10 grams total fat, 2.5 grams saturated fat, 0 grams trans fats, 75 milligrams cholesterol, 63 milligrams sodium, 20 grams carbohydrates, 2 grams fiber, 15 grams sugars, 24 grams protein.

MUSHROOM CHILI

Chef Richard Perry opened his first restaurant in St. Louis in 1970 and is considered a pioneer in U.S. cooking, with a national reputation for culinary prowess. His latest venture is EatPlan, a personal chef business that provides sensible portions of great Midwestern American cookery to help promote good health. His meatless chili will appeal to even die-hard carnivores. This is a Countdown USA Recipe.

2 cloves garlic, minced
1 medium onion, chopped
3 stalks celery, chopped
½ pound mushrooms, sliced
1½ green peppers, chopped
1 tablespoon extra-virgin olive oil
1 tablespoon water
2 sixteen-ounce cans unsalted tomatoes, diced
2 sixteen-ounce cans kidney beans, drained
3 tablespoons chili powder

1. Sauté the vegetables in the oil and water until tender.
2. Add the remaining ingredients. Cover and cook over low heat for 1 hour, stirring occasionally.

Serves 6

Nutritional info per serving: 170 calories, 4 grams total fat, <1 gram saturated fat, 0 grams trans fats, 69 milligrams cholesterol, 276 milligrams sodium; <1 gram carbohydrates, 1 gram fiber, 3 grams sugars, 27 grams protein.

SNAPPER WITH GOLDEN TOMATO SALSA AND MELON-JICAMA RELISH

Chef Stephan Pyles helped put Southwestern cuisine on the national map with his restaurants Routh Street Café, Baby Routh, and Star Canyon. He received the 1991 Best Chef Award–Southwest from the James Beard Foundation. In this recipe, Pyles uses snapper, but you can use any firm white fish to make a delicious healthful meal. This is a Countdown USA Recipe.

Salsa
1 pound ripe yellow tomatoes, peeled, seeded, and diced
2 tablespoons diced red bell pepper
2 tablespoons diced green bell pepper
2 tablespoons minced fresh chives
2 serrano chilies, ribbed, seeded, and minced
1 tablespoon fruit vinegar (such as raspberry or orange)
salt (if desired) and pepper to taste
1 tablespoon chopped fresh cilantro

Relish
1 mango, peeled and pulp removed
1 serrano chili, ribbed and seeded

1 tablespoon lime juice
1½ tablespoons finely diced (⅛") red bell pepper
¾ cup diced (¼") cantaloupe
½ cup diced (¼") honeydew melon
2 tablespoons peeled, seeded, and diced (¼") cucumber
½ cup peeled and diced (¼") jicama
2 tablespoons chopped fresh cilantro
salt (if desired) to taste
pepper

Fish
¼ cup unsaturated oil (olive, canola, safflower, or corn oil)
4 snapper fillets, 6–8 ounces each
flour for dredging

Salsa
In a large bowl, combine the tomatoes, bell peppers, chives, and serrano chilies. Toss and season with the vinegar, salt (if desired), pepper, and cilantro. Set aside.

Relish
1. In a food processor, puree the mango, serrano chili, and lime juice.
2. Add the remaining ingredients and puree. Season to taste. Set aside.

Fish
1. Heat the oil in a skillet until slightly smoking.
2. Season the fish on both sides. Dredge in flour.
3. Sauté 2–3 minutes per side.
4. Serve with the salsa and relish.

Serves 4

Nutritional info per serving: 403 calories, 17 grams total fat, 3 grams saturated fat, 0 grams trans fats, 102 milligrams cholesterol, 200 milligrams sodium, 8 grams carbohydrates, 1 gram fiber, 54 grams protein.

GRILLED BREAST OF CHICKEN WITH SPRING VEGETABLES AND VERMOUTH

Chef Marcel Desaulniers co-owns The Trellis restaurant in Williamsburg, Virginia. He is the author of several cookbooks, including *Death by Chocolate* and *Desserts to Die For,* and has earned the Best Chef–Mid-Atlantic Region Award from the James Beard Foundation. His chicken entrée takes less than 30 minutes to prepare. This is a Countdown USA Recipe.

2 tablespoons fresh lemon juice
2 tablespoons dry white wine
salt to taste (optional)
pepper
4 four-ounce boneless, skinless chicken breasts
¼ pound snow peas, trimmed
½ pound shelling peas, shelled
¼ pound asparagus, stems trimmed, peeled
1 medium carrot, cut into 2½" × ⅛" strips
¼ cup vermouth
1 small red onion, thinly sliced
1 tablespoon safflower oil (or other unsaturated oil)
1 medium tomato, peeled, seeded, and chopped
¼ pound mushrooms, stems trimmed, sliced ⅛" thick

1. Combine the lemon juice, white wine, salt (if desired), and pepper. Sprinkle over the chicken breasts.
2. Wrap each chicken breast separately in plastic wrap and refrigerate.

3. Blanch the vegetables separately as follows in boiling water, then drain and refrigerate.

snow peas—20 to 30 seconds

shelled peas—20 to 30 seconds

asparagus—45 seconds

carrots—1½ minutes

4. Grill the chicken over a medium hot charcoal or wood fire, or broil for about 1½ minutes on each side.

5. Transfer the chicken to a baking pan. Pour the vermouth over the chicken and cover lightly with foil.

6. Bake the chicken in a 350° oven for 10 minutes.

7. Sauté the onion in the oil for 1 minute. Add the peas and carrot and sauté for 1 minute. Add the tomato and asparagus and sauté for 2 minutes. Add the mushrooms and sauté for 1–2 minutes.

8. Divide the vegetables into 4 servings. Place each serving on a plate. Place 1 chicken breast on each plate of vegetables. Serve immediately.

Serves 4

Nutritional info per serving: 200 calories, 5 grams fat, 1 gram saturated fats, 0 grams trans fats, 70 milligrams cholesterol, 104 milligrams sodium, 8 grams carbohydrates, 2 grams fiber, 4 grams sugars, 30 grams protein.

VEGETABLE AND SIDE DISHES

Vegetables are filled with fiber and flavor that can help you feel full on fewer calories. They're naturally low in calories, so take advantage of them to make a leaner plate. When you don't deep-fry vegetables, even potatoes can be a healthy choice.

DELICIOUS OVEN FRIES

Adapted from *Keep the Beat: Heart Healthy Recipes,* by the National Heart, Lung, and Blood Institute.

Who says you can't have fries? These fries are spicy and flavorful and don't come with the unhealthy trans-fatty acids found in most commercially prepared fries. Tip: Mix the vegetable oil with the spices to evenly coat the fries, rather than brushing on the oil after the fries are in the pan. Use a nonstick pan and place the pan on the lowest rack of your oven so that the fries are less likely to stick to the pan.

ice water
4 large russet potatoes (about 2 pounds), scrubbed
1 teaspoon garlic powder
1 teaspoon onion powder
¼ teaspoon salt
1 teaspoon ground white pepper
¼ teaspoon ground allspice
1 teaspoon dried hot pepper flakes
1 tablespoon vegetable oil (olive, canola, safflower, corn, or peanut oil)

1. Fill a large bowl with ice water.
2. Scrub the potatoes. Cut in half lengthwise, then into ½" strips. Under cool running water, rinse the potatoes to remove starch, then place them in the ice-water bath. Let them sit for 60 minutes or longer to chill thoroughly (if making ahead, cover and refrigerate).
3. Meanwhile, combine the other ingredients in a resealable plastic bag.
4. Place the oven rack on the lowest position. Preheat the oven to 475°.

5. Remove the potatoes from the ice water and pat dry with paper towels. Place the potatoes in the bag with the spices and oil and shake to coat evenly. Spread the potatoes in a single layer on a nonstick baking sheet.

6. Cover the sheet with foil and bake for 15 minutes. Remove the foil and continue baking, turning the fries occasionally until golden brown, 15–20 minutes more.

Serves 5 (1 cup per serving)

Nutritional info per serving: 238 calories, 4 grams total fat, 1 gram saturated fat, 0 grams trans fats, 0 milligrams cholesterol, 163 milligrams sodium, 48 grams carbohydrates, 5 grams fiber, 5 grams protein, 796 milligrams potassium.

SMOTHERED GREENS

Adapted from *Keep the Beat: Heart Healthy Recipes*, by the National Heart, Lung, and Blood Institute.

Whether you live south of the Mason-Dixon Line, where cooked greens are a staple, or north of it, this is a wonderful, flavor-filled recipe to add to your cooking repertoire because it is loaded with nutritious ingredients, from potassium to folic acid. Traditionally, smothered greens come loaded with unhealthy fat, but not this version. Note: Two pounds of greens may seem like a lot, but they cook down quickly to 4 or 5 servings. Smoked turkey gives these greens great flavor, but if you're going vegetarian, you could use smoked tofu, tempeh, or other meat substitutes as alternatives. If you're not counting milligrams of sodium, add salt to taste.

2 pounds greens (about 18 cups packed; mustard, turnip, collard greens, or kale, or a mixture)
3 cups water

1 tablespoon chopped red chili peppers (may substitute a few
    drops of hot pepper sauce such as Tabasco)
¼ teaspoon cayenne pepper
¼ teaspoon ground cloves
2 cloves garlic, crushed
½ teaspoon dried thyme
1 scallion, chopped (both white and green parts)
1 teaspoon ground ginger
¼ cup chopped onion
¼ pound skinless smoked turkey breast, roughly chopped
salt to taste (optional)

1. Wash the greens thoroughly in cool water, making sure to get rid of any sand or grit. Remove and discard the stems and dry the greens slightly with paper towels. Tear the greens into bite-size pieces and set aside.

2. In a large pot over high heat, bring the water to a boil and add the remaining ingredients except the salt. Once the mixture has come to a boil, add the greens. Stir to incorporate the seasonings and reduce the volume of greens, about 1 minute.

3. Reduce the heat to low and cook, uncovered, for 20–30 minutes, or until the greens are tender. Add salt as desired to taste. Before serving, discard the garlic, if desired.

Serves 5 (1 cup per serving)

Nutritional info per serving: 80 calories, 2 grams total fat, <1 gram saturated fat, 0 grams trans fats, 16 milligrams cholesterol, 378 milligrams sodium, 9 grams carbohydrates, 4 grams fiber, 9 grams protein, 472 milligrams potassium.

RICE PILAF

Recipe courtesy of Emeril Lagasse.

1 tablespoon unsalted butter
¾ cup chopped yellow onion
1 cup long-grain white rice
1¾ cups canned low-sodium chicken broth, or chicken stock
½ teaspoon salt, to taste
2 tablespoons thinly sliced green onion (optional)

1. Preheat the oven to 350°F.
2. Melt the butter in a large ovenproof saucepan or Dutch oven over medium-high heat. Add the onions and cook, stirring, until soft, about 3 to 4 minutes. Add the rice and cook, stirring until opaque and nutty in aroma, 2 to 3 minutes. Add the chicken broth and salt, stir well, and bring to a boil. Cover with a tight-fitting lid and transfer to the oven. Bake until the rice is tender and the liquid is absorbed, about 25 to 30 minutes.
3. Remove the rice from the oven and let stand for 5 to 10 minutes. Fluff the rice with a fork and stir in the green onion, if desired. Serve hot.

Serves 4

Nutritional info per serving: 220 calories, 4 grams total fat, 1 grams saturated fat, 0 grams trans fats, 3 milligrams cholesterol, 35 milligrams sodium, 48 grams carbohydrates, 1 gram fiber, 6 grams protein.

PASTA

Pasta is a fast food that also has a long shelf life, so it's a great staple to keep in your pantry. Because it's a dehydrated food, pasta—even white pasta—does not raise blood sugar as much as many other processed foods, such as white bread. So if you can't stomach whole grain, go ahead, have regular pasta. Just watch portion sizes and add plenty of healthy toppings to make it a well-rounded meal.

SUMMER VEGETABLE SPAGHETTI

Adapted from *Keep the Beat: Heart Healthy Recipes,* by the National Heart, Lung, and Blood Institute.

Serve this vegetarian pasta dish hot or cold.

2 cups small yellow onions, cut in eighths
2 cups (about 1 pound) ripe tomatoes, peeled and chopped
2 cups (about 1 pound) yellow (summer) and green (zucchini)
squash, thinly sliced
1½ cups (about ½ pound) fresh green beans, cut
⅔ cup water
2 tablespoons fresh basil or cilantro, minced
1 clove garlic, minced
¼ teaspoon salt
black pepper to taste
½ teaspoon chili powder
1 six-ounce can tomato paste
1 pound spaghetti, uncooked (white or whole wheat)
½ cup Parmesan cheese, grated

1. In a large saucepan, combine the onions, tomatoes, squash, green beans, water, basil or cilantro, garlic, chili powder, salt, and black pepper. Cook for 10 minutes, then stir in the tomato paste.

Cover and cook for 15 minutes, stirring occasionally, until the vegetables are tender.

2. Cook the spaghetti in unsalted water according to package directions.

3. Spoon the sauce over the drained hot spaghetti. Sprinkle Parmesan cheese on top.

Serves 9 (1 cup spaghetti with ¾ cup sauce with vegetables)

Nutritional info per serving: 271 calories, 3 grams total fat, 1 gram saturated fat, 0 grams trans fats, 4 milligrams cholesterol, 328 milligrams sodium, 436 milligrams potassium, 51 grams carbohydrates, 5 grams fiber, 11 grams potassium.

RED HOT FUSILLI
Adapted from *Keep the Beat: Heart Healthy Recipes,* by the National Heart, Lung, and Blood Institute.

1 tablespoon olive oil
2 cloves garlic, minced
¼ cup fresh parsley, minced, plus extra for garnish
4 cups chopped ripe tomatoes
1 tablespoon fresh basil, (chopped or 1 teaspoon dried)
1 tablespoon oregano leaves, crushed (or 1 teaspoon dried)
¼ teaspoon salt
ground red pepper or cayenne to taste
½ pound chicken breasts, cooked, diced into ½" pieces, or ¾
    pound if raw (optional)
8 ounces uncooked fusilli (or try a combination of whole wheat and
    white pasta, but cook whole wheat and white pasta separately)

1. Heat the oil in a medium saucepan. Sauté the garlic and parsley until golden.

2. Add the tomatoes and spices. Cook uncovered over low heat for 15 minutes, or until thickened, stirring frequently. If desired, add the cooked chicken and continue cooking for about 15 minutes, or until the chicken is heated through and the sauce is thick.

3. Cook the pasta in unsalted water until firm but not soft (al dente).

4. Spoon the sauce over the pasta and sprinkle with coarsely chopped parsley. Serve hot as a main dish or cold as a side dish or lunch.

Serves 4 (1 cup per serving)

Nutritional info per serving (without chicken): 293 calories, 5 grams total fat, 1 gram saturated fat, 0 grams trans fats, 0 milligrams cholesterol, 168 milligrams sodium, 489 milligrams potassium, 54 grams carbohydrates, 4 grams fiber, 9 grams protein.

Nutritional info per serving (with chicken): 391 calories, 8 grams total fat, 1 gram saturated fat, 0 grams trans fats, 48 milligrams cholesterol, 211 milligrams sodium, 629 milligrams potassium, 54 grams carbohydrates, 4 grams fiber, 27 grams protein.

ITALIAN SAUSAGE PASTA

Used by permission of the Whole Grains Council and Oldways Preservation Trust.

8 ounces whole wheat spiral pasta

2 links Italian chicken or turkey sausage, or vegetarian "sausage," crumbled into small bits

2 cups mixed chopped veggies—your choice (such as red peppers, zucchini, onion, mushrooms, broccoli, garlic)

1 teaspoon olive oil

1 cup cleaned chopped spinach

1 25-ounce jar unsweetened spaghetti sauce
freshly grated Parmesan cheese (optional)

1. Fill a large saucepan with water and bring it to a boil. Add the pasta and cook according to package directions.
2. Brown the sausage bits in a nonstick skillet until cooked through and golden outside.
3. Sauté the chopped veggies in the olive oil until tender-crisp.
4. Add the spinach, spaghetti sauce, and sausage to the veggies and warm until the spinach wilts.
5. Drain the pasta and combine with the sauce-veggie-sausage mix. Top with Parmesan cheese, if desired.

Serves 4

Variations
- Choose different vegetables.
- Substitute leftover chicken, beans, or shrimp for the sausage.

Nutritional info per serving: 430 calories, 8 grams total fat, 1 gram saturated fat, 0 grams trans fats, 25 milligrams cholesterol, 1,518 milligrams sodium, 72 grams carbohydrates, 5 grams fiber, 19 grams sugars, 22 grams protein.

SPAGHETTI SAUCE
Made from nearly fat-free ground turkey and lean ground beef, this spaghetti sauce is high in protein. Courtesy of Holly Edelbrock, Allison Shircliff, and Barbara Burke of the Clinical Research Center at the University of Washington, www.crc.washington.edu. Used by permission.

8 ounces raw 10 percent fat ground beef
20 ounces raw 99 percent fat-free ground turkey
4 teaspoons olive oil

1⅛ cups tomato paste
2 teaspoons onion flakes
2 teaspoons sugar
2 teaspoons garlic, minced
¼ teaspoon black pepper
¼ teaspoon Italian seasoning
2 cups water
1½ tablespoons grated Parmesan cheese

1. Sauté the meat and oil over medium or medium-high heat until browned and thoroughly cooked. Add the rest of the ingredients to the meat. Stir all ingredients together until well mixed.

2. Lower the heat to medium low and simmer for 20 minutes, stirring occasionally.

Serves 8

Nutritional info per serving: 215 calories, 7 grams total fat, 3 grams saturated fat, 0 grams trans fats, 49 milligrams cholesterol, 159 milligrams sodium, 13 grams carbohydrates, 3 grams fiber, 28 grams protein.

DESSERTS/SNACKS

APPLE COFFEE CAKE
Adapted from *Keep the Beat: Heart Healthy Recipes*, by the National Heart, Lung, and Blood Institute.

5 cups tart cored, peeled, chopped apples (such as Granny Smith)
1 cup sugar (or 1 cup Splenda or a combination of sugar and Splenda)

1 *cup dark raisins*

½ *cup pecans, chopped*

¼ *cup vegetable oil (canola, sunflower, safflower, corn, or olive)*

2 *teaspoons vanilla extract*

1 *egg, beaten (or equivalent egg substitute)*

2 *cups all-purpose flour, sifted (if you can, try to make it whole wheat white flour for more nutrition and fiber; King Arthur Flour, www.kingarthurflour.com, produces a whole wheat white flour from winter white wheat with all the nutritional benefits of darker whole wheat flour)*

1 *teaspoon baking soda*

2 *teaspoons ground cinnamon*

1. Preheat the oven to 350°.

2. In a large mixing bowl, combine the apples, sugar, raisins, and pecans. Mix well and let stand for 30 minutes. Stir in the oil, vanilla, and egg.

3. Sift together the flour, baking soda, and cinnamon. Stir into the apple mixture about a third at a time to slowly moisten the dry ingredients.

4. Turn the batter into a 13" × 9" × 2" nonstick pan. Bake for 35–40 minutes. Cool the cake slightly before serving.

Serves 20 (serving size is about 3½" × 2½")

Nutritional info per serving: 196 calories, 8 grams total fat, 1 gram saturated fat, 0 grams trans fats, 11 milligrams cholesterol, 67 milligrams sodium, 136 milligrams potassium, 31 grams carbohydrates, 2 grams fiber, 3 grams protein.

FROSTED CAKE

Who said you can't have your cake and eat it, too? This cake has a hint of orange, and the cocoa can help satisfy a chocolate craving.

Adapted from *Keep the Beat: Heart Healthy Recipes,* by the National Heart, Lung, and Blood Institute.

Cake
cooking oil or nonstick cooking spray
2¼ cups cake flour
2¼ teaspoons baking powder
4 tablespoons margarine (without trans-fatty acids)
1¼ cups sugar
4 eggs (or equivalent amount of egg substitutes)
1 teaspoon vanilla extract
1 tablespoon grated orange peel
¾ cup skim milk

Icing
3 ounces low-fat cream cheese
2 tablespoons skim milk
6 tablespoons cocoa
2 cups confectioners' sugar, sifted
½ teaspoon vanilla extract

Cake
1. Preheat the oven to 325°.
2. Grease a 10" round pan (at least 2½" high) with a small amount of cooking oil or use nonstick cooking oil spray. Powder the pan with flour. Tap out the excess flour.
3. Sift together the flour and baking powder.
4. In a separate bowl, beat together the margarine and sugar until soft and creamy. Beat in the eggs, vanilla extract, and orange peel. Gradually add the flour mixture, alternating with the milk, beginning and ending with flour.
5. Pour the batter into the prepared pan. Bake 40–45 minutes, or until done. (A toothpick inserted in the middle should come

out clean.) Let the cake cool 5–10 minutes before removing from the pan. Let cool completely on a wire rack before icing.

Icing

1. Cream together the cream cheese and milk until smooth. Add the cocoa and blend well.

2. Slowly add the sugar until the icing is smooth. Mix in the vanilla extract.

3. Smooth the icing over the top and sides of cooled cake.

Serves 16

Nutritional info per serving: 241 calories, 5 grams total fat, 2 grams saturated fat, 0 grams trans fats, 57 milligrams cholesterol, 273 milligrams sodium, 95 milligrams potassium, 45 grams carbohydrates, 1 gram fiber, 4 grams protein.

1-2-3 PEACH COBBLER

Adapted from *Keep the Beat: Heart Healthy Recipes,* by the National Heart, Lung, and Blood Institute.

½ teaspoon ground cinnamon
1 tablespoon vanilla extract
2 tablespoons cornstarch
1 cup peach nectar
¼ cup pineapple juice or peach juice (or use juice reserved from canned peaches)
2 cans (16 ounces each) sliced peaches, packed in juice, drained (or 1¾ pound fresh peaches, peeled and sliced)
1 tablespoon tub margarine (without trans fats)
nonstick cooking spray (as needed)
1 cup dry pancake mix

⅔ cup all-purpose flour (whole wheat white if possible)
½ cup sugar
⅔ cup evaporated skim milk
½ teaspoon almond extract
½ teaspoon nutmeg
1 tablespoon brown sugar

1. Preheat the oven to 400°.

2. Combine the cinnamon, vanilla, cornstarch, peach nectar, and pineapple or peach juice in a saucepan. Cook over medium heat, stirring constantly, until the mixture thickens and bubbles.

3. Add the sliced peaches. Reduce the heat and simmer for 5–10 minutes.

4. In another saucepan, melt the margarine (or melt in microwave). Set aside.

5. Lightly spray an 8" square glass dish with cooking spray. Pour the hot peach mixture into the dish.

6. In another bowl, combine the pancake mix, flour, sugar, and melted margarine. Stir in the milk. Quickly spoon this over the peach mixture. Add the almond extract.

7. Combine the nutmeg and brown sugar. Sprinkle on top of the batter.

8. Bake for 15–20 minutes, or until golden brown.

9. Cool and cut into eight pieces.

Serves 8

Nutritional info per serving: 271 calories, 4 grams total fat, <1 gram saturated fat, 0 grams trans fats, <1 milligram cholesterol, 263 milligrams sodium, 284 milligrams potassium, 54 grams carbohydrates, 2 grams fiber, 4 grams protein.

POWER-PACKED PEANUT BARS

These tasty bars don't require baking and cost less than the energy or cereal bars that are commercially available. Recipe courtesy of the National Peanut Board (www.nationalpeanutboard.org).

> 2 cups toasted rice unsweetened ready-to-eat cereal (such as Rice Krispies)
> ½ cup dried, unsweetened fruit (raisins, cranberries, blueberries, mangoes, your choice)
> 2 cups rolled oats
> ¾ cup chopped peanuts
> ½ cup peanut butter (creamy or crunchy, or substitute almond, cashew, or other nut butter if you prefer)
> ½ cup firmly packed brown sugar
> ½ cup light corn syrup
> 1 teaspoon vanilla extract

1. In a large bowl, mix together the cereal, dried fruit, oats, and nuts. Set aside.

2. Place the peanut butter, brown sugar, and corn syrup in a small saucepan over low heat or in a microwavable container. On the stovetop, stir constantly over medium heat until the mixture is smooth and just starts to boil. Then microwave on high for about 2 minutes. Stir so the mixture is smooth.

3. Stir in the vanilla.

4. Pour the liquid mixture over the cereal. Gently toss to mix well and coat the cereal with the liquid ingredients.

5. Pour the mixture into a nonstick 8" or 9" square baking pan (8" if you want squares, 9" if you want bars). Press so that the mixture is even and level. Cool completely. Cut into 12 squares or bars. Wrap each bar individually in plastic wrap. Store in an airtight container or freeze.

Makes 12 squares or bars

Nutritional info per square/bar: 265 calories (depending on ingredients), 10 grams total fat, 2 grams saturated fat, 0 grams trans fats, 0
milligrams cholesterol, 65 milligrams sodium, 39 grams carbohydrates, 3 grams fiber, 24 grams sugars, 8 grams protein.

CHOCOLATE CHEESECAKE

Yes, you really can indulge with this high-protein, low-fat recipe,
courtesy of Holly Edelbrock, Allison Shircliff, and Barbara Burke
of the Clinical Research Center at the University of Washington,
www.crc.washington.edu. Used by permission.

8 ounces fat-free cottage cheese, blended until smooth
¾ cup unsweetened cocoa powder
5 ounces low-fat cream cheese, softened
14 ounces fat-free cream cheese, softened
1½ cups Splenda
⅛ cup sugar
6 large egg whites
2 teaspoons vanilla extract
2½ tablespoons chocolate fudge ice-cream topping

1. Preheat the oven to 300°.
2. Combine all the ingredients except for the chocolate topping. Whip until creamy.
3. Place the batter in 10 large custard cups, or 10 large muffin
tins, or a springform pan sprayed with Pam or other healthy oil
spray. Place into a hot-water bath and bake for 30 minutes or until the top starts to crack.
4. Remove from the oven and let cool. Spread with chocolate
topping. Refrigerate.

Serves 10

Nutritional info per serving: 250 calories, 6 grams total fat, 2 grams saturated fat, 0 grams trans fats, 15 milligrams cholesterol, 335 milligrams sodium, 31 grams carbohydrates, 2 grams fiber, 19 grams protein.

SMOOTHIE

Research from Barbara Rolls, Ph.D., Pennsylvania State University professor of nutrition and author of *Volumetrics,* shows that this kind of high-volume breakfast has a lot of staying power.

The smoothie is a good source of calcium, protein, and fiber—depending what fruit is used. Berries, for example, are high in fiber.

1 cup nonfat plain yogurt
½–1 banana (depending on taste preferences and calorie goals)
½ cup fruit (fresh or frozen)
2 ounces unsweetened cranberry juice
1–1½ cups ice cubes
1 teaspoon vanilla (optional)
Splenda to taste (optional)
1 teaspoon honey (optional)

1. Place the yogurt, banana, additional fruit, and cranberry juice in a blender or food processor. Mix until smooth.

2. Add the ice and blend until smooth and thick. Tip: The longer you blend the smoothie, the more air it contains, which increases volume and helps you feel full with fewer calories.

3. Add the optional ingredients, if desired.

4. Pour into a glass and get a straw. Or put into a container to drink on the way to work.

Serves 1

Nutritional info per serving: 293 calories, 1 gram total fat, 0 grams saturated fat, 0 grams trans fats, 5 milligrams cholesterol, 192 milligrams sodium, 59 grams carbohydrates, 4 grams fiber, 44 grams sugars, 16 grams protein.

MANGO SHAKE

A refreshing drink or snack that is also rich in potassium, one nutrient that many Americans fail to eat enough. You can use any frozen, unsweetened fruit.

Adapted from *Keep the Beat: Heart Healthy Recipes,* by the National Heart, Lung, and Blood Institute.

2 cups low-fat or skim milk
4 tablespoons frozen mango juice, unsweetened (or a fresh
*   mango, pitted and cut into chunks, frozen)*
1 small banana, cut into chunks, frozen
2 ice cubes

Put all the ingredients into a blender or food processor. Blend or pulse until foamy. Add more ice as needed. Serve immediately.

Serves 4 (¾ cup per serving)

Nutritional info per serving: about 106 calories (depending on fruit used), 2 grams total fat, 1 gram saturated fat, 0 grams trans fats, 5 milligrams cholesterol, 63 milligrams sodium, 361 milligrams potassium, 20 grams carbohydrates, 2 grams fiber, 5 grams protein.

INDEX OF RECIPES

INDEX